Navy SEAL
BREAKTHROUGH TO
Master Level
Fitness™

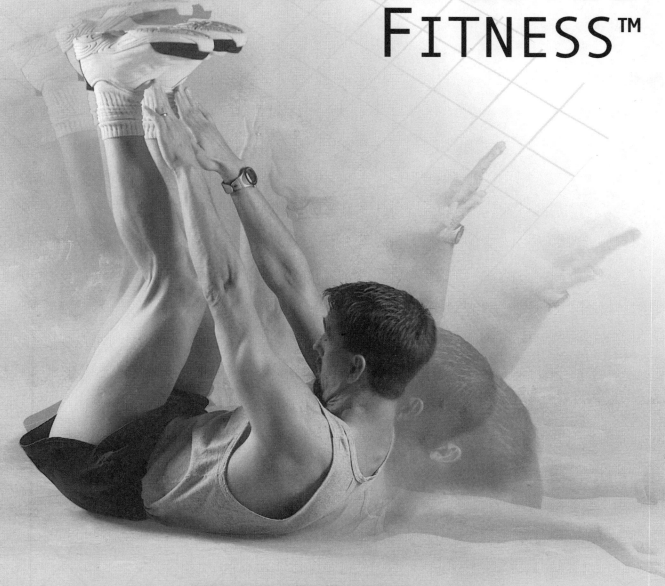

NAVY SEAL
BREAKTHROUGH TO
MASTER LEVEL
FITNESS™

The Ultimate Training System
to Irresistible Strength &
a Body-to-Die-For

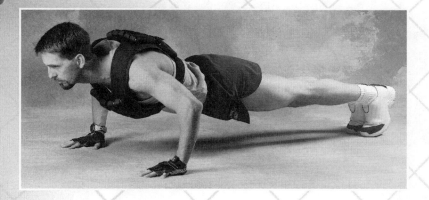

MARK De LISLE

Strength
& Honor

BRONZE
BOW PUB

Disclaimer

The exercises and advice contained within this book may be too strenuous or dangerous for some people, and the reader should consult a physician before engaging in them.

The author and publisher of this book are not responsible in any manner whatsoever for any injury that may occur through reading and following the instructions herein.

Published by Bronze Bow Publishing, Inc.
2600 East 26th Street, Minneapolis, MN 55406.
You can reach us on the Internet at www.bronzebowpublishing.com.

Literary development and cover/interior design by
Koechel Peterson & Associates, Inc., Minneapolis, Minnesota.

Manufactured in the United States of America.

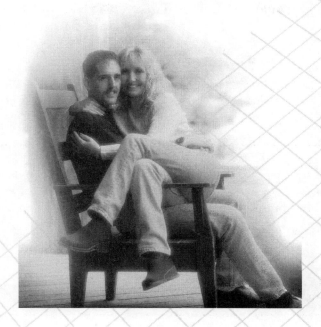

determination and excellence

DEDICATION

This book is dedicated to all UDT/SEALs, past and present, who have given true meaning to the words *determination* and *excellence*.

Also, to my beautiful and loving wife Wendy, who is my inspiration and reason for living. You have been there to support me in every trial and every goal. You will always have my heart. To this day you never stop to amaze me. My fins off to you, babe!

And to my kids, who suffered so much while I was training away from home. I love you, Mark and Michelle. You are the reason why I gave up active duty. We lost many years due to me being away from home, and I will never be able to return those years. Remember always that each day is a new page, and we can make of it how we want. I will always carry each of you in my heart.

To Melissa, Lacey, Jed, and Dax, change is never easy, but life places obstacles in front of us for growth. We all have had to learn to compromise, adjust, and tear down walls. I am so glad that you have come into my life. All of you have seen your mom and me work hard to give you a foundation of love, respect, and faith. Never forget that I will always be there for you.

CONTENTS

INTRODUCTION

Whether it's stepping up your workout to Master Level Fitness or making it through the SEAL's infamous Hell Week, I am writing to tell you that you can do it. I know you can, and I say this for many reasons, which will follow in the book, but I start with my personal story. I want to give you more than just advice on fitness and motivation by clarifying where I am coming from in life. My point here is that *I did it—and so can you.*

> Being proactive is more than taking initiative. It is recognizing that we are responsible for our own choices and have freedom to choose based on principles and values rather than on moods and conditions. Proactive people are agents of change and choose not to be victims, to be reactive, or to blame others.
> —Stephen R. Covey

Trust me, my life has not always been this way. I grew up living the American dream—supportive parents, good neighborhood, good school, Little League—until the early '70s when my father's career began to have well-deserved success. Unfortunately, my parents did not cope well with that success, and their priorities went astray. Out of respect for my parents, I wish to keep the details private. Let's just say that my parents were not always in control

I sit here at my desk on a quiet Saturday night with much reflection. My wife and kids are away visiting relatives, and I've finished writing most of this book. I try to keep busy, but my thoughts keep returning to how grateful I feel to be where I am today. Living in a peaceful neighborhood where friends watch out for one another, I have a roof over my head, and, best of all, I have a wife whom I love deeply and who loves me equally. I never dreamed I could experience a relationship so filled with peace, security, mutual respect, and love. My whole world could fall apart around me, but I know that Wendy will always be at my side to support me.

of their lives, and I was exposed to things no child should experience. And being the eldest child, I caught the brunt of most of it. By my junior year in high school, I was basically on my own. My mother was still there, but she was having trouble just trying to survive and make ends meet. In my senior year I had to give up wrestling and baseball to work and pay for school clothes.

For years I was told I was good for nothing and would never amount to anything. Constantly reminded about how inadequate I was, I began to feel very insecure, always looking for recognition but never finding it. Though I loved football and truly wanted to excel at it, my father said I was too small and not good enough to play. This became the issue that triggered my desire to take on challenges.

Even though I was only a freshman and needed to be a sophomore to get into weight-lifting class, I pleaded with the coach and wouldn't take no for an answer. I soon began to lift weights, and by my junior year I was one of the strongest athletes in my school. I had speed and loved the challenge of going one-on-one, so the position of wide receiver peaked my attention. I ended up making all-conference my senior year and achieved goals far beyond my own expectations.

That was one of the many challenges I met as a young man on my own. Some challenges I overcame, and others I made mistakes with and ended up getting beat. One of those regarded my need for companionship. When I was twenty-one, I met a sweet nineteen-year-old girl who was as naive as I was. We thought that marriage would solve all our problems and make us happy. We soon had a reality check, and after four years of struggling we divorced and hoped to at least keep our friendship intact. Once again, I was left feeling lost and a failure.

With no self-esteem or direction in my life, I took my father's advice and joined the Navy. I hoped they could give me a life foundation to build upon. While in boot camp, I saw a film called "Be Someone Special," which was a recruit-

ing tool for the Navy SEALs. I didn't know what a Navy SEAL was, but for the first time in my life I realized I had the opportunity to take on a challenge that no one could keep me from accomplishing but myself. After around three hundred of us tried out in boot camp, two of us qualified to go to BUD/S.

My father was upset that I was giving up the electronics training I originally signed up for, and he and the rest of my family, feeling I'd never make it, pretty much wrote off the idea. But even though no one else around me believed in me, *I did*, and that was all that mattered. Yes, I was out of shape, skinny, and small, but inside I had the desire of a panther. Once I got going, I knew that nothing could stop me. Inner desire and determination are tremendous gifts that few of us fully learn how to tap into, but I was learning.

What a tremendous experience SEAL training was for me! Although it was the most difficult thing I had ever experienced in life, I would not be where I am today if it wasn't for the SEAL Teams. Training at an extremely grueling pace, at times I wondered when it would end. Of course, driving nine hours one way to see my kids in Sacramento on the weekend twice a month when I should have been resting didn't help. But my kids mean the world to me, and it was well worth it. Phase by phase, I made it through and finally made it to the dream—I became a member of SEAL Team Three!

> With no self-esteem or direction in my life, I took my father's advice and joined the Navy. I hoped they could give me a life foundation to build upon. While in boot camp, I saw a film called "Be Someone Special," which was a recruiting tool for the Navy SEALs.

The bonds of friendship I formed in the SEALs and the lessons I learned will last a lifetime. In the SEAL teams you are valued and judged by the load you carry and how much you put out. Not by what title you carry or how much money you have. What a difference it would make if that value system was carried over into the workplace and in life. This is something we plan to implement in our fitness boot camp for executive training and individuals. Think of the power and influence of an executive or manager who leads and guides his co-workers by personal example and ethical principles rather than by wielding an office title.

Life's challenges did not stop when I left active duty. Though I left so I could be with my kids again, my father, who initially called me an idiot for joining the SEALs, now railed against me for leaving. And when my ex-partner RJ Wolf and I decided to self-publish the first edition of *Navy SEAL Exercises*, my family and friends thought I was crazy to try it without any experience or knowledge of the publishing industry. But by now I was so practiced in relying on my own self-worth that I had the extra strength I needed.

Knowing that we had an exercise routine that would change the industry, I went for it. With no advertising budget, no experience in marketing, advertising, or public relations, we took the book to a best-seller level. We sold over 60,000 copies

> **What a tremendous experience SEAL training was for me! Although it was the most difficult thing I had ever experienced in life, I would not be where I am today if it wasn't for the SEAL Teams.**

and got appearances on *Crook & Chase, CNN, Extra, Outside* magazine, *Exercise for Men Only, Navy Times,* and many more. The President of the United States even ordered copies. I am proud of the many lives it has touched and the changes it brought to those people and the fitness industry. Now six years later, boot camp workouts are the rage, and people are getting back to basics again. Obviously, others jumped on the bandwagon with more assets and marketing dollars, but I never did it for the money in the first place. I just hope it helped some people find their true potential.

With our limited assets, in 1998 RJ and I knew that we were not going to be able to support each other and achieve the income levels we wanted to achieve if we remained partners. What we did not realize was that our budget was so tight that even the monthly payment that was made to buy RJ out would put *SEAL Fitness* out of business. Funds had to be taken out of advertising to make payments, resulting in fewer book orders, which snowballed for everything else. *SEAL Fitness* lasted just a few short months after this. Though $30,000 in debt and feeling panicked, I was able to utilize the talents I had acquired as a SEAL to get a job as the Director of Corporate Relations and Sales at the American Council on Exercise (ACE). I started to make payments on the old debts and glimpsed light at the end of that tunnel. Then I met Wendy, and life looked so much better. We knew instantly that we were meant for each other, and just a short two months later we were married. The CEO of ACE was sympathetic to my situation and allowed me to move to Utah, since Wendy lived there, and work out of a home office.

But life loves to throw kinks my way. Little did I know that one month after I moved everything to Utah the CEO of ACE would quit. The new CEO came onboard from Reebok and immediately asked, "What is my Sales Director doing in Utah?" I was soon given the choice to pack up and move again or lose my job. But I was not about to let a career choice get in the way of my new family. I found myself living in the rural community of Torrey, Utah, population five hundred, with no work, no income, a new family, and a load of debt. Once again, I dug deep into my SEAL training and recalled that whatever I put my mind to I can accomplish.

Today, three and a half years later, I live near Park City, Utah, with my family happy and

> You can use this book to help yourself feel better, stronger, healthier, centered, and focused. It is out there. You just have to go get it!

settled, a new book in the works, a job as the Director of Corporate Relations for Gold's Gym in this region, and the amazing possibility of having my fitness camp finally up and running next year. All debt with *SEAL Fitness* has been paid off except for a few minor accounts. Wendy and I are now in the process of building our first home together and couldn't be happier in our marriage. A rewarding life—emotionally, physically, and spiritually—which seemed but a distant dream is now my reality.

Stephen Covey reminds us that we can be proactive or reactive in life. I choose to be proactive and take charge of my life. I still make mistakes, but I am growing and learning. That's my word to you: Be proactive with your life. Take the time to evaluate where you are going, what you want out of life, and how you can get there. Sometimes the methods and manners that you choose to accomplish your goals are more important than actually accomplishing them. Take this time to change your life.

1

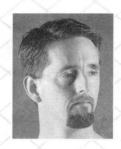

" Find this fire, bring it to the surface, and harness its power for your workouts. *"*

MENTAL TOUGHNESS

As more and more press has been released on the Navy SEALs over the past few years, the entire world has become aware of how extraordinary these men are. I have never found another group of men so dedicated to their fields and their lives as my fellow frogmen of the SEAL Teams. I have the highest and utmost respect for them, and for this reason I wish to help civilians in all walks of life capture their drive, their zeal for life.

Let's face it! Not everyone can become a frogman, but everyone can find that same determination in his or her life, particularly as it relates to physical fitness. Our self-worth . . . our spirit . . . our inner fire is what drives us every day to go after what we want out of life. In the SEAL Teams we called it *fire in the gut*. Some days it is stronger than others, and some days it seems as though

there is nothing there. My purpose in this section is to help you find this fire, bring it to the surface, and harness its power for your workouts. Without it, you might as well use this book to light your fire in the fireplace, because that is all it is worth—the paper and ink.

Consider how easily we humans are sparked. Something as simple as a commercial on television can get us to yell and scream. A song on the radio can trigger emotions totally unrelated to what we've been thinking. The piercing sound of a police siren instantly cuts loose an adrenaline rush. Of course, a few seconds later we simmer back to normal. What we need to do is discover what fires you up and how to keep it going.

If your personal motivation for exercising is simply to look good, you're not going to get far.

You need to go deeper and find out for yourself why you are working out and why you want this. Hopefully your list will include finding a healthier lifestyle, living a longer, meaningful life, sleeping better, feeling better, and, of course, looking better. While these are only a few suggestions, the key is for you to attach your goals and motivation to multiple reasons. When you get beyond the superficial and find true motivation, you will find your personal *fire in the gut*. Each of us has it, it's really there, but we experience it to different degrees. Now we just have to yank on it a little so that you can experience this phenomenon, and once you do you'll get addicted to it—in a positive way of course. When fatigue, stress, and mental blocks kick in, the *fire in the gut* is what says get back up and go again.

By way of example, in the winter of 1999 I watched my wife's high school wrestling team take on Dixie High School. Wayne High School was supposed to dominate every match. There was a lot of emotion that night because an ex-pupil of Wayne's coach was now the Dixie head coach. In every match the Wayne wrestler came out fired up, but after the first period each one gave up mentally, physically, and emotionally. Dixie High School completely dominated the entire meet, and Wayne went home defeated in front of their home crowd. I teasingly asked my wife what had happened to her so-called "championship team," but I knew right away what had happened and exactly what this team needed.

I presented myself to head coach Kerry Anderson and asked if I could experiment with the team by exposing them to some unorthodox training methods. My intent was to give them a watered-down version of SEAL training, which the team did not know as Coach Anderson intro-

duced me to the team. As the team members looked my way, I could see it in the young men's eyes: "What is this old man doing here? Does he think he is going to work me over?" I explained that I did not care who they were or who they thought they were, but I expected 110 percent and perfect technique. I told them, "Look, I don't care if you can do 200 push-ups and 200 sit-ups. In my training sessions you will do exactly as I say and perform the exercises exactly as I demonstrate." I tried to let them know that the strength and repetitions will come along slowly, but no one can use bad techniques and receive optimal results.

We began the routine to a chorus of snickers. The boys kept asking, "Why are we stopping at two pull-ups and then two push-ups?" As the routine progressed, the voices stopped and the wincing and groaning began. By the time we finished one hour later, every kid was face first into the mat and not moving. I said, "Guys, your transformation is beginning, and if you trust me your fitness levels will reach new heights." As the season progressed, I watched these freshmen and sophomores change, and along with their physical changes came an attitude transformation. They quickly learned that the human body will go far beyond what they thought it could. Their minds became a strength rather than a weakness, and these young kids went on as ninth and tenth graders to become state champions.

I'd like to give special thanks to Coach Anderson as well as to all the boys for letting me experiment. Fins off to Randy Morrell (three-time state champion), KC Anderson, Gavin Pace, Rhett and Dallas Edwards, and the gang—you showed your *fire in the gut* and proved the effectiveness of this workout routine.

2
THE TRUE MEAN-
ING OF FITNESS

When it comes to personal fitness, most of us look first to the quick fix. We want immediate results, and we'd like them to be dramatic! But the reality is that there is no quick fix, and there is no program or plan out there that can transform us into Arnold or Sly in two weeks. Both of them will tell us that it took years of hard work and sweat to get to the level they reached.

My philosophy is that anything worth obtaining in this life, anything of real value, involves sweat, hard work, and lots of dedication. If getting into great physical shape came easy for us, we would not appreciate the results in the same manner as someone who has worked hard to achieve the same goal. The fact is that personal fitness always requires a change of lifestyle that involves dealing with our emotions, exercise, diet, and sleeping habits. Our purpose here is to give you quick and easy tools that will help you achieve this change.

To achieve Master Level Fitness, all that I ask from you is three to five days a week, 45 to 90 minutes per routine. I am not proposing that you work out seven days a week and two hours a day. You won't get there by beating yourself to death. Far too many of us set well-intentioned goals, but those goals are so high that they end up beating us up constantly. We purpose that in two weeks we will lose twenty pounds and five inches in the waist. Then at the end of two weeks we look in the mirror, shake our head in disgust, and say, "Forget this. I haven't changed one bit. This will take forever."

In order for fitness to become a successful part of your life, it must first become a way of life for you. I am well aware that it will involve a struggle. To be perfectly honest, there have been periods when I've compared my ultimate personal fitness goals with where I was at the moment, and I stopped working out. I had to force myself to get off the couch and push my body to move. But once I started conditioning and hit my tenth workout, it became a habit again. I have found that the secret to staying motivated and fired up is to always compare where you were when you started to change your life and where you are now rather than where you want to get to.

When I say that fitness must become a lifestyle, here's how you make it work. Don't look at your goals for a year from now but rather what you want to specifically accomplish this week and day. For instance, you may say to yourself, "Today I want to pyramid to seven exercise repetitions instead of six, and by Friday I am going to cut ten seconds off my run time." If you add up that seemingly small increase of one repetition and ten seconds over a period of six months, the change becomes significant. Take one day at a time, and soon this whole process of transforming becomes simple.

Take a good look at your life and determine what you like and dislike about it. Make a list of the pros and cons of your current conditioning, eating habits, time dedicated to exercise, and overall self-worth. Take all your pros and use them as guidelines for your goals. Next, take all your cons and arrange them into a list of priorities from top to bottom. Determine that you are going to take one con each month and turn it into a strength. Notice that I said you will work on one per month, not the whole list. For example, if one of your cons is that you never get out of the house to run or walk, set your resolve that on two days this week you will run or walk. Two weeks later, resolve to run or walk three days, and so on.

As far as your pros, let's say you put down that you have managed to cut down on your fat intake. Your next goal might be to target for elimination the excessive sodas you've allowed in your weekly diet. As simple as this may sound, it leads to another positive change in your fitness lifestyle. We had a saying in the SEAL Teams that applies here: "KISS"—"keep it simple, stupid." You do not need to reinvent yourself in this process, but just keep modifying your way to success.

I also want you to write down *everything* you eat for an entire week, and I mean anything that goes in your mouth. You will be amazed at how much food your body is consuming. Once you have a clear picture of your weekly food intake, you can begin to accurately and intelligently modify your diet. We all make mistakes when it comes to controlling our eating habits, and we do not need to become Mr. or Mrs. Nutrition 101 in order to correct them.

Diet is such a key factor in your success. It can have a major effect on your recovery time, energy levels, and progression in the areas of stamina, strength, and performance. Do not underestimate this part of your routine and transformation. Critiquing my own diet has been an invaluable addition to my workout program, and every so often I find myself needing to retune it. If you take the new awareness learned from this test and add to it the enthusiasm that you get from starting any new routine, I guarantee that you will see the value of putting more effort into what your body needs and

what it actually intakes. For more information, look to the Nutrition section at the back of the book.

One other major factor when it comes to the meaning of fitness regards your sleep. Over the last ten years, experts have raised sleep to nearly the top of the list of importance for a successful exercise routine. Few of us realize just how much sleep deprivation, excessive stress, and our daily living environment can play havoc with our bodies. Sleep is one of the best antidotes for our day-to-day trials. The person who thinks he can go all day, push an exercise routine, and survive on four or five hours of sleep a night is setting himself up for a crash. Eventually something in the body is going to give and then shut down. It could be the heart from stress, or the stomach from ulcers, or just about any other malady.

Whether it regards the hours we commit to sleeping or to our lives in general, we must set the priorities for our lives and then live them out practically. Remind yourself that we live in a society so driven to get ahead that millions sacrifice their families and themselves all the time. Some have reached the pinnacle of success in the business world, but at a tremendous personal cost. It may not be work-related, but all of us have our life issues to prioritize. As much as I loved the SEAL Teams, I had to decide whether I would train for nine months out of the year or be with my family. It was an extraordinarily difficult choice, but my family had to be my highest priority.

Get your life priorities straight and make fitness a dynamic part of it. Then put your heart into your workouts and do it for the right reasons. Don't let the reason for exercising be because everyone will compliment how good you look or in order to be with a certain someone who requires that you maintain a certain look. Make fitness a constant part of your lifestyle by doing it for yourself . . . and no one else.

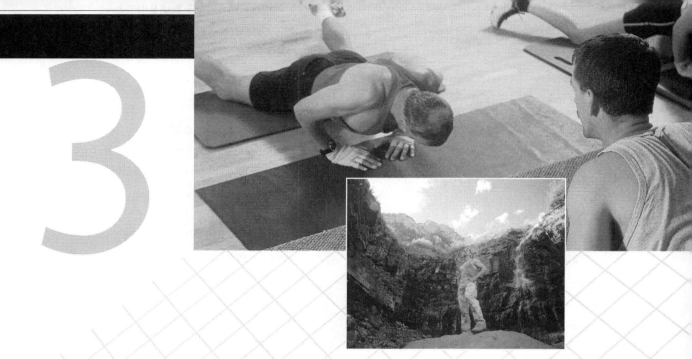

3

What this will give you
is a nicely chiseled
triathlete build.

CHOOSING THE CORRECT
PROGRAM FOR YOU

Different exercise routines give different results, and these results will affect whether you stick with it. To best describe what *Mark De Lisle's Navy SEAL Breakthrough to Master Level Fitness* routine is going to do for you, I compare it to a triathlete program. It is going to increase your endurance, stamina, strength, muscle tone, and muscle density. Make no mistake: you are not going to come out of this looking like Steve Goldberg or Lou Ferrigno. *This is not a body-building exercise program*, but what it will give you is a nicely chiseled triathlete build.

If you are a female, I hope you do not get scared off by the phrase "Navy SEAL Exercises." There is such a prevailing misconception today that if women exercise or lift weights they will end up looking as though they are competing for Ms. Olympia. That is not what our routine does. You are going to tone and build muscle, which in turn will increase the amount of calories your body burns. The end result is less body fat and a sculptured look that you have trained to acquire.

The *Master Level Fitness* routine is designed to teach you to improve your overall conditioning level. You cannot spot reduce, but you can improve specific areas of your body by exercising the entire body. Remember: the goal is to improve the overall conditioning level of your entire body.

Which leads me to another area of concern. Many people think that if they go to the gym and lift weights for an hour they are in great shape. I have taken some of these so-called "gym junkies" and put them through a calisthenics routine with a nice two- or three-mile run afterward and watched them fizzle. Even though they had improved their overall strength levels, they had no cardio-conditioning, and thus their overall

fitness levels were low. They have trained for quick-burst energy, but they need sustained strength. I personally love to lift weights, but there is so much more to fitness than just weights. Resistance training improves bone density, muscle tone, joint mobility, and calorie burning, but don't equate that with overall fitness. I want you to be able to have an active lifestyle at sixty or seventy years of age. I want you to run and not be weary, to walk and not faint, and this routine can do it for you.

You can combine this program with your current weight-lifting regimen. For example, if you decide to work your chest and triceps one day, then you can utilize the push-up and bar dip routines as your first set prior to free weights. If you are going to work the back and shoulders, then utilize the pull-up routine as the first set prior to weights. And after you have finished your leg routine, take off on a good run or sprinting session. Always remember the importance of stretching after a good warm-up and after your routines. Some of your best gains in flexibility will come after you have finished exercising.

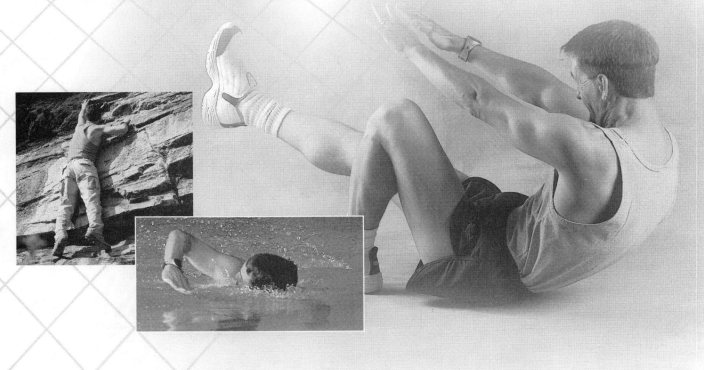

4

GOAL SETTING

Setting realistic, measurable goals for exercise programs is often overlooked or treated lightly. Some people get away without being clear about their objectives, but I have seen many others become demoralized or even quit their routines because they were not satisfied with the results. It actually wasn't that they were not getting results, but their expectations of miracles in short periods of time had crumbled. You are not going to be transformed in 30 days. You are not going to drop 50 pounds and have a rock hard body. But you can expect to see changes and drop weight.

Remember that this program is going to cut your body fat, increase your strength, improve your performance, and boost your energy levels. But simple logic tells you that muscle weighs more than fat. So if you increase your muscle mass while cutting your body fat, is your weight going to drop any significant amount? Probably not. It is a mistake to worry about weight rather than to concentrate on measurements and performance.

You need to create a fitness log that allows you to record measurements, cardio-conditioning, heart rates, exercise performance, and, yes,

if you wish, weight. Start out with the following measurements.

1. Neck
2. Shoulders
3. Biceps (flexed)
4. Chest (relaxed, flexed)
5. Waist
6. Hips (females)
7. Thigh
8. Calves

Our cardio measurements can be broken down into times in sprinting distances, long distance, swimming, and so on. Heart rate can be broken into two categories: resting and maximum heart rate. The best time to figure out your resting heart rate is while you are still lying in bed from a good night's rest. Without even stepping onto the floor, take your heart rate. To determine your maximum heart rate, perform an exercise, such as stair climbs, as fast as you can for 2-3 minutes. Then take your pulse, repeating the exercise two or three times to calculate the average.

Exercise performance is just a matter of writing each exercise on a piece of paper and breaking them into categories of 30, 60, 90, and 120 day intervals. With the abs you should write down how many reps you can perform in complete sets from one end of the routine to the other. At any given time someone can probably perform hundreds of sit-ups or leg raises, but what we are concerned about is if you can perform 30 of each exercise all the way through the full blitzing routine. When it comes to the pyramid system, use the peak of the pyramid as your tool for measurement (for instance, 2-4-6-4-2).

Do yourself a favor and be realistic when it comes to goals that you wish to accomplish. Stating that you will drop 40 pounds and 20% of your body fat in 30 days is to guarantee failure. A far better goal would be to break down the loss of 40 pounds and 20% of your body fat over a twelve-month period. That is both realistic and obtainable.

So do the math. 40 pounds divided by 12 months = 3.33 pounds. 20% body fat divided by 12 months = 1.66%. Next, divide these goals by weeks. 3.33 pounds divided by 4 weeks = .83 pound. 1.66% body fat divided by 4 weeks = .415% of your body fat. Now, these are obtainable goals. You don't concentrate on the 40 pounds and 20% of your body fat. Keep your focus on the .83 pound and .415% of your body fat per week. Don't get caught up in weighing and measuring on a daily basis. Just pick one day a week or even one day every two weeks for checkups. You will stay much more relaxed and focused on your task at hand.

Keep your goals in visual range. We humans tend to be very visual. Post your weekly goals in key locations to be seen on a daily basis, i.e., mirrors, refrigerators, car dashes, and doors. Wherever you need the motivation to stay

focused and fired up, keep your goals in front of your eyes. By achieving your weekly goals, you will get results you want because the long-term goals will come naturally.

And reward yourself for accomplishing your goals, especially the long-term ones. Determine your rewards ahead of time. When you reach your long-term goals, give yourself a trip or something to fit the new you. Husbands or wives, maybe it's something you have desired for a long time. Make it simple and easy but enough to pat yourself on the back. It really helps to attach rewards to accomplishments. They can be key tools in motivation when you feel lazy and want to skip your routine. By the way, reaching short-term goals does not warrant rewarding yourself with an ice cream sundae and thereby negating the loss. Never allow a reward to be counterproductive.

I guarantee that if you do not go into this program with a plan or goals, you will not get everything you expect out of it. Goals keep us focused, driven, and satisfied. Do not take them lightly, and do not wait until you are two months into the program to set goals for yourself. You need the measurements, performance levels, and goals to keep yourself on track.

If you apply these same principles to the other areas of your life as well, it can be transforming. Whether it regards your career, your personal relationships, your intellect, or your spiritual life, goals provide a path for improvement. No one is ever perfect, but there is no reason to not strive to be the best we can. Just understand that we all make mistakes along the way. When you fall down, wipe off the dirt and apply what you've learned to avoid making the same mistake again. Goals will help you to do so.

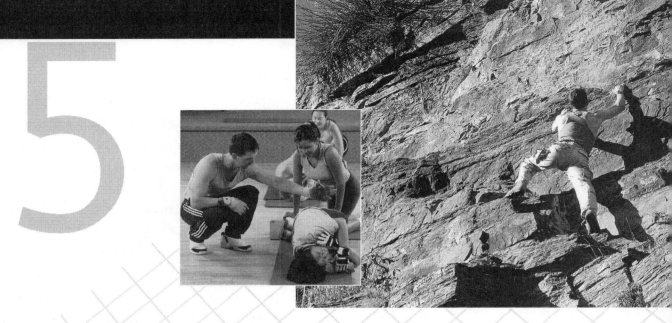

5

You must push the limits of your
body—mentally, physically,
and emotionally.

LET'S GET TO WORK

Throughout this book I will not speak to you as though you are a first year medical student or weary you with long explanations of why a muscle contracts and relaxes. What you will find is basic instructions that are easy to follow and to the point. I have learned over the past years that most people just want a proven program that they can effectively put to work for themselves.

We have tried this routine on thousands of customers and military personnel, all with amazing results. I am thrilled to pass you this tool that has worked marvelously for me, but what you do with it really depends upon you. If you want it to work for you the way it is intended, your goal must be perfect technique. And you must push the limits of your body, but not beyond what is considered physically safe. Each of you will deter-

mine what those limits are, but unless you push your limits, why even start a program?

Now let's get to work! Take a full sheet of paper and a pencil and write out your year-long fitness goal. Next, break that exact goal down into monthly and then weekly goals. Use this to create a graph that shows how much weight you want to lose over the year, each month and week, and then break it down one more time to a daily weight loss. Use this sheet of paper as your goal chart and display it in an easily accessible location where you can see the progress you are making. If you make a daily target your main focus, this simple one-day goal will change your life!

Use this same principle and apply it to your exercise levels and achievement goals. As each day passes, I want you to go to your goal chart and check off your accomplishment. Do not worry about your monthly and yearly goals, because as you check off your daily and weekly goals, the rest will naturally fall into place. You can completely avoid the overwhelming sensation of how you are going to lose twenty pounds when your goal is one pound at a time.

With your goals ready to go and in plain sight, now you need to find out your fitness level.

FITNESS EVALUATION

I want you to take each exercise in this book and perform a fitness evaluation. Here's how it works. Using push-ups as an example, perform as many regular push-ups in one set as you can, going to the point of exhaustion. Take your total number of repetitions and write it down on your goal sheet. Let's say you can perform a maximum of 110 push-ups. We will now utilize the pyramid system to determine the peak of your pyramid, which is where you should start. Add $2 + 4 + 6 + 8 + 10 + 12 + 14 + 12 + 10 + 8 + 6 + 4 + 2 = 98$. When you can reach within + or - 10 from the total max, then you have found the start point.

Your pyramid can be lowered or raised to find the optimum starting point. Perhaps you can only do 110 push-ups maximum, but you have great endurance. Which means that pyramiding up to 14 to start just does not quite give you the burn you need. Obviously then, you need to increase your starting pyramid to 16. The same principle is true for someone who has great quick-start energy but little endurance. You may have to lower your starting point to 12. The goal is to receive a good burn on the backside of your pyramid—$12 + 10 + 8$ and so on.

When it comes to pull-ups, use regular pull-ups as your guide. For example, you can do a total of 30 regular pull-ups. Take the pyramid system again: $2 + 4 + 6 + 8 + 6 + 4 + 2 = 32$. With pull-ups you can adjust your routine by + or - 2. 8 pull-ups should be the peak point of your pyramid.

Use this same method for formulating all your upper body routines, but the formula for working your abs is slightly different. For your abs, divide your maximum output of sit-ups by 3, and this will give you the number to begin your ab routine. For example, if your maximum is 125 sit-ups total, then your fitness routine will be in the 40 reps per exercise range. A good recommendation for a time frame for your test is 2 minutes (you can also apply this time limit to push-ups and pull-ups). This way you are not sitting on your back resting while trying to squeak out those 25 extra reps. This test is a test of exhaustion. As noted before, you can adjust this evaluation to fit your body type. You may have to increase or decrease your routine by + or - 5.

You now have your goals set, and your routine levels dialed in. We are ready to concentrate on technique and make this program work. Good luck, stay focused, and do not break technique for reps.

I cannot overemphasize that you need to be medically cleared to begin this program. If you are fighting any previous injuries, it is better to let them properly heal, or you may be fighting a lifetime of ailments. If at any point in this routine you feel a muscle pulling, stop immediately, then ice it down for 20 minutes on and 20 minutes off. It is not worth it to overexert yourself and pull a muscle. Take it slow and stay within your means. An injury can also affect your enthusiasm, keep you from continuing on with the routine, or limit your success.

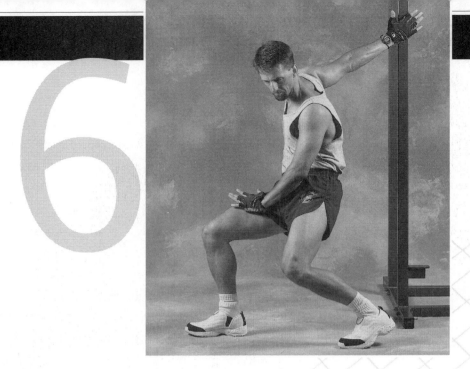

6

One of the most important elements of your fitness

STRETCHING

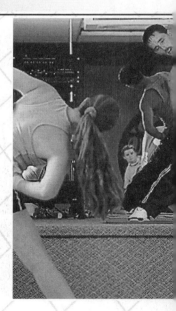

Stretching is one of the most important elements of your fitness routine. If you take the time to warm up for at least five minutes and then follow it with a full body stretching program, your results will far exceed your own expectations. I also recommend that you stretch in between every third exercise within each routine to maintain pliability in your muscle tissues. When muscles are pushed to their peak performance, they tighten and lose their optimal levels. By relaxing and allowing your muscle group to take a short break and stretch, you will improve the effectiveness of your routine, and your muscle fiber output will increase.

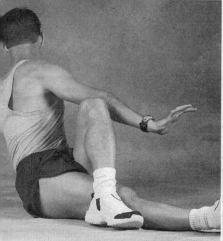

outine.

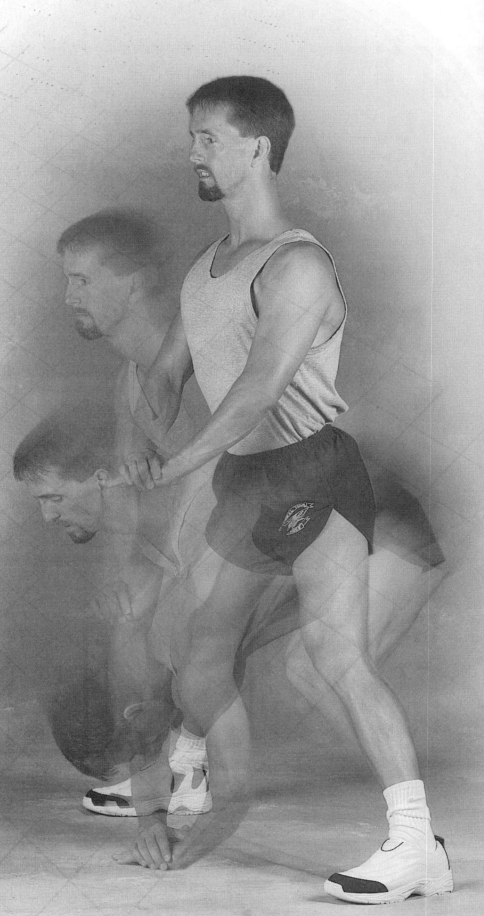

t c h

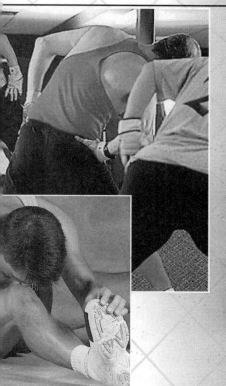

WARM-UPS

When beginning any exercise routine, remember that warm-ups and stretching are two separate entities. Warm-ups allow you to increase muscle temperatures, and they deliver oxygen to your muscle while increasing blood flow. Compare it to taking a piece of meat out of the refrigerator and trying to stretch it. If you allow it to reach room temperature, it will stretch farther. By warming up, you are going to prevent injuries. These same techniques apply to running or swimming. It is recommended that you spend some time jogging at a slow pace prior to stretching for running, or swimming at a slow pace prior to stretching for swimming.

JUMPING JACKS

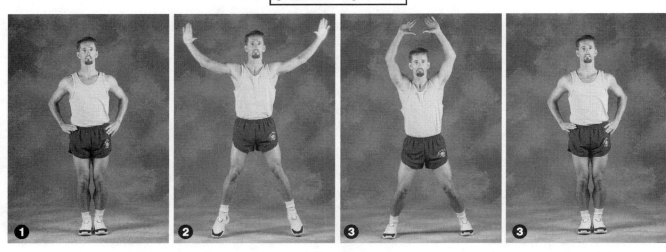

FIGURE 1 Hands by your side, feet together.

FIGURE 2 Light thrust, using your lower body as you rise to the balls of your feet. Lightly extend your hands above your head while spreading your feet to more than shoulder-width apart all in the same motion. Touch your hands as they join.

FIGURE 3 Lower hands back down to your sides as you bring your feet back to their original position.

Warm-ups and stretching are two separate entities.

HALF JUMPING JACKS

This warm-up is much quicker with shorter movements. Half Jumping Jacks are similar to Jumping Jacks except that while Jumping Jacks take one second to complete one repetition, Half Jumping Jacks take half a second to complete one repetition. Keep your movements smooth and fluid to prevent injury.

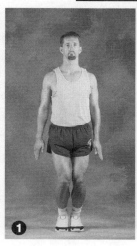 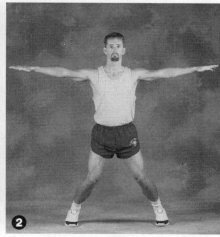 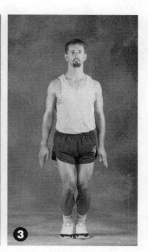

FIGURE 1 Hands by your side, feet together.

FIGURE 2 Once again, rise to the balls of your feet. With one smooth thrusting motion, jump up as you bring your hands to a 45° angle, while spreading your feet more than shoulder-width length.

FIGURE 3 Bring your feet and hands back to the starting position.

RUNNING IN PLACE

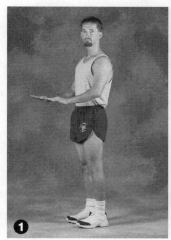 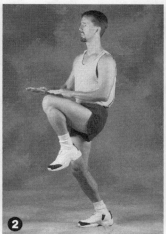 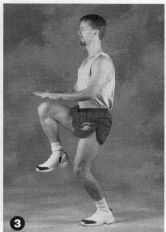

What distinguishes these warm-ups is that you are going to place your arms at a 90° bend with palms facing downward. This forces you to hit your hands each time you raise a knee and not slack off. Keep in mind that this is a warm-up, not a race, and you are not intended to push it beyond a nice jog. You may wish on your own to incorporate this warm-up as an exercise by increasing the intensity and difficulty later on.

FIGURE 1 Standing straight up, place arms at 90° bend with palms facing down.

FIGURE 2 Starting with your left leg first, raise your left knee to the point that it touches your left hand. Repeat the same action to your right knee.

FIGURE 3 The following is how the warm-up looks in sequence.

STRETCHES

Stretching needs to be an integral part of your fitness routine, and without it your gains will be limited. Not only do you halt your progress, but you leave yourself open to injuries. Do not take this section lightly or just spend a few minutes on it. Stretching should be approached in the same manner you give to your upper or lower body workouts.

Take your time and perform each stretch with perfect technique. Do not concern yourself with how limber you are. This is a great time to get in tune with your body and learn how to listen to it. As you stretch you will find that your body has varying points of discomfort. It is important to push yourself to this point of discomfort but not beyond. Once the sensation turns from discomfort to pain, you are pushing your muscle fibers too far. Keep in mind that your greatest gains in flexibility will come in your stretching session at the *end* of your routine.

BEND OVERS

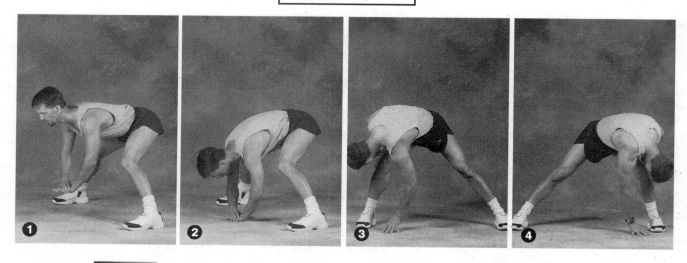

FIGURE 1 Place your hands together out in front of you. As you bend over, keep your shoulders back and your lower back straight. Pushing your chest forward while performing this stretch will help keep your lower back straight.

FIGURE 2 As your hands come close to the floor, take a deep breath and exhale all the air from your lungs. At this point let your body go limp. You will notice in general that you will be able to increase your stretch by at least an inch if done properly. This will allow you to reach your optimal position for the stretch. If lowering your hands to the floor is not enough, continue lowering yourself to your elbows.

FIGURE 3 Now place your right hand on the back of your right calf. Lower yourself back down and touch your right foot with your left hand. Press your chest against your knee. You may need to use your right hand on the floor to maintain your balance.

FIGURE 4 Perform the exact same motion as in Figure 3 but to the opposite foot.

CROSS OVERS

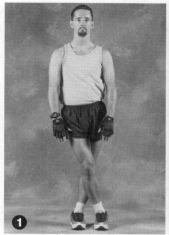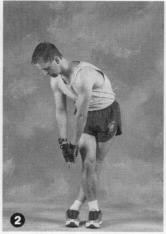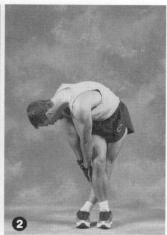

This particular stretch is very beneficial to the back, the knee, the hamstrings, and the outside of your knee.

Figure 1 Standing straight up with your hands by your side, cross your right foot over your left foot.

Figure 2 As you begin to lower your upper body, twist it to the right so that your hands touch the inside of your left calf.

Perform the same motion but to the opposite leg.

INNER THIGH STRETCH WITH MODIFICATION

This stretch is excellent for the inner thighs, but we have added a modification to get more out of it.

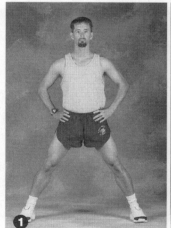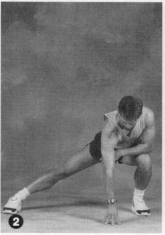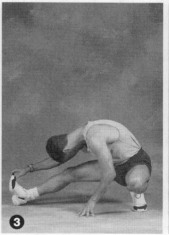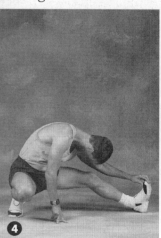

Figure 1 With your feet flat on the ground, spread them apart so that they are slightly farther than shoulder width.

Figure 2 As you lean to your left, place your left elbow on your left thigh. Take your right hand and place it on the ground as a balance point. Now lean to the left or right as far as you can without pulling your feet off the ground.

Figure 3 This is the modification. Once you have reached your 15 seconds in the stretch position, drop down so that you are sitting on your heel. Reach over and grab your right toe. Slowly pull yourself down to your right knee.

Figure 4 Repeat steps in Figure 3 but to your opposite leg.

FORWARD LUNGE STRETCH

The most common mistake with lunges is not stepping out far enough. The forward lunge stretch is a good stretch if your hip flexors are tight on your upper thighs. The key is to place the right forearm on the thigh of your right leg as you stretch forward. Place your opposite hand on the ground for balance. Take this stretch slow and easy. The important part is to find that point where the muscle tightens, then go slowly beyond that.

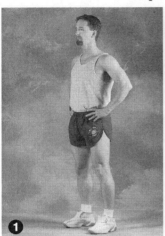 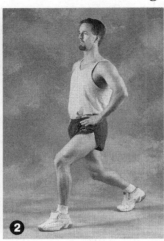 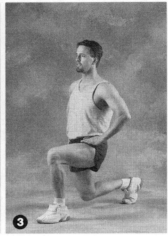 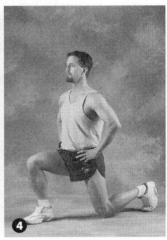

FIGURE 1 Stand with your feet together and your hands on your hips.
FIGURE 2 Step forward with your left leg to the point that you have 3-3 ½ feet between your feet.
FIGURE 3 Lower your right knee to the ground and create a 90° bend in the left leg. Once again place your right arm or forearm on the thigh of your right leg. As your knee is fixed on the ground, begin to slowly move your entire body forward to stretch the thigh and hip flexor.
FIGURE 4 Repeat the process with your left leg.

SIDE AND OBLIQUE STRETCH

This particular stretch is a good stretch for the obliques and the lats.

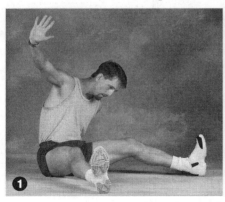 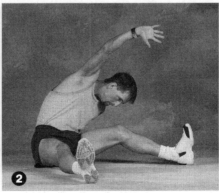 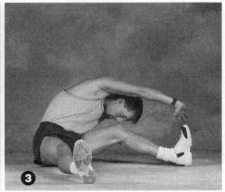

FIGURE 1 Sit down and spread your legs so that they are more than shoulder-width apart.
FIGURE 2 While left hand is behind your hip, place your right hand above your head and begin leaning toward your left knee.
FIGURE 3 Try to reach with your left foot to make this stretch successful. Maintain your arm above your head. Repeat the steps in Figure 2 but to your opposite leg.

HAMSTRING STRETCH

This next stretch is actually a very common but effective stretch. Where we modify it is in the legs. We found that over the years added stress is placed in the knee area by locking your legs in the straight position. By slightly bending your knees, you will alleviate this stress.

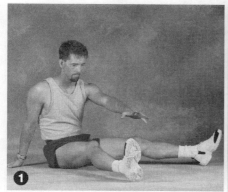 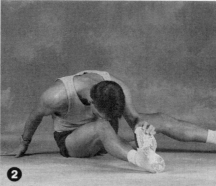 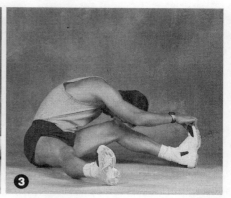

FIGURE 1 Place your legs in a good V formation with your right hand placed slightly behind your hip.

FIGURE 2 Place your left hand on the tips of your toes of your right foot. A little helpful hint as you become more flexible; place your hands lower down the bottoms of your shoes. Push off your right hand while pulling with the left.

FIGURE 2 Bring your chest down to your knees and maintain this position for about 10-15 seconds. Next, relax and return to the original position.

FIGURE 3 Switch sides and repeat the process.

HURDLER STRETCH

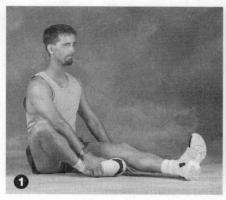 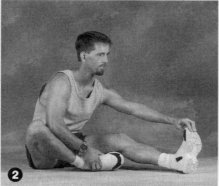 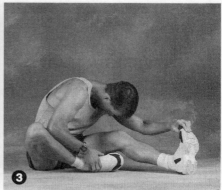

FIGURE 1 Sit down and bring your right foot next to your left knee so that the inner sole is flat against the leg.

FIGURE 2 Grab your left foot with your left hand while placing your right hand underneath your right foot. Place your right elbow into your right calf or knee. Keep the right knee as low as possible while stretching your left hamstring.

FIGURE 3 Try to touch your chest to your left knee. Switch legs when finished.

BUTTERFLY

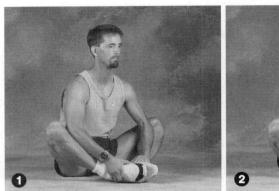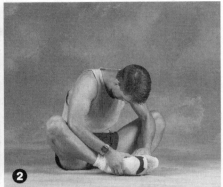

FIGURE 1 While sitting down, place your hands underneath your outside ankles. Place your elbows into your knees or calves.

FIGURE 2 In one fluid motion, begin pressing your knees down to the ground as you pull up with your hands. As you do this, begin to lean forward with your upper body.

ITB STRETCH

This stretch is terrific for runners. As you pull your knee toward the chest, you will feel the entire side of your leg begin to stretch. This is where you will find the ITB tendon (Iliotibial). This stretch also helps to loosen up your lower back. Do not be afraid to bear hug this position. Second recommendation is to wrap your left arm around the lower shin, then squeeze. This should cause your right foot to rise off the ground.

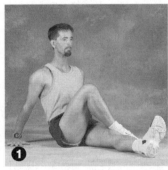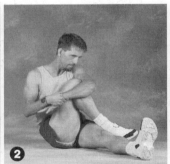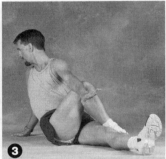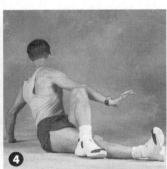

FIGURE 1 While sitting down, place your right foot on the outside of your left knee.

FIGURE 2 Wrap your left arm around your lower right shin. Squeeze your right knee tightly against your chest and hold for 15 seconds. Your right foot should rise off the ground from the squeeze. Do not be afraid to squeeze tight.

FIGURE 3 Place your left elbow on the outside of your right knee. Next, place your right hand about a foot behind the middle of your back. Once in this position, begin to rotate your right shoulder to the right while pushing your right knee to the left. It is very important to look straight back while performing the stretch.

FIGURE 4 Repeat on the opposite side.

This is the perfect stretch to really see how breathing affects your results. When you reach the optimal point of your stretch, I want you to take in a deep breath, then exhale it all. As you reach the end of your exhale, try to stretch just a little bit more. Let your entire upper torso go limp.

SITTING THIGH STRETCH

This is one of those stretches you do not want to rush.
Take your time getting into position as well as returning to the start position.

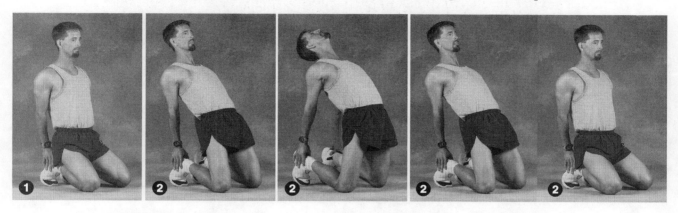

FIGURE 1 While sitting on your heels, place your hands on your heels.

FIGURE 2 Lift your hips upward as you pull your shoulders back. Relax and allow this stretch to work. At the peak of this stretch you should be on the tips of your toes. Once you have finished, slowly lower your hips back to your heels.

CALF STRETCH

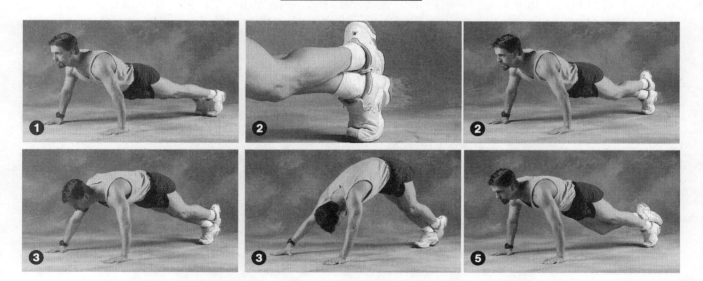

FIGURE 1 Start in the regular push-up position.

FIGURE 2 Place your left leg over your right leg crossing at the ankles.

FIGURE 3 Raise your buttocks straight in the air until your legs and arms reach a 45° angle.

FIGURE 4 Repeat the exercise with the opposite leg crossed.

STANDING THIGH STRETCH

With the standing thigh stretch, your technique can make or break the effectiveness of the stretch. Most exercise enthusiasts stand upright when they perform this stretch, but if you bend over at the hips it will dramatically change the stretch. You must continue to pull your foot toward your lower back even as you bend over.

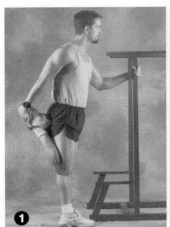 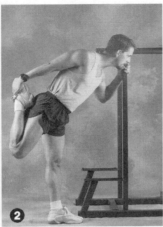 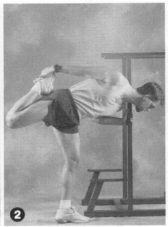 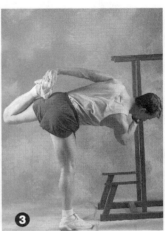

FIGURE 1 Grab a solid object or pole that will allow you to maintain balance throughout the stretch. Next, grab your foot by placing your hand on the top section of your foot.

FIGURE 2 Begin to pull your foot toward the lower back.

FIGURE 3 Slowly bend over until your upper body is in a 90° position. As you begin to bend over, you will begin to feel the tension in the your thighs.

LAT STRETCH

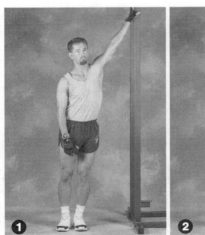 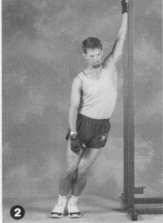 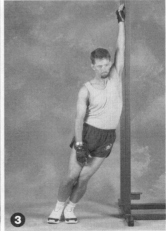

FIGURE 1 Place yourself sideways against the wall. Step away from the wall at least one to two feet.

FIGURE 2 Reach as high as you can with your left hand.

FIGURE 3 Once you cannot reach any higher, drop down to the point that your left elbow touches the wall. As your elbow touches the wall, bend your knees and continue lowering. Repeat to the opposite side.

CHEST STRETCH

The key to this stretch is the placement of your hand on the wall. You need to have your hand with the palm facing sideways and the fingers away from your body. The height of your hand can make or break this stretch. If your hand is too low, you are stretching just the shoulders. You must have the hand placed slightly higher than your shoulders. Play with this one until you get the exact position you need to stretch the chest along with the shoulders. Do not forget to bend your knees to get into proper position.

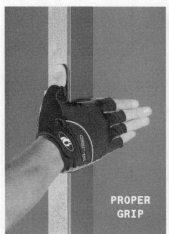 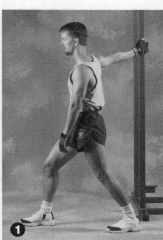 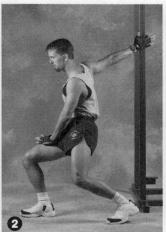 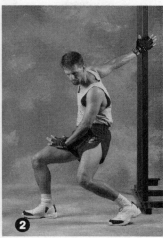

PROPER GRIP

FIGURE 1 Stand sideways against a wall. Place your right hand on the wall with the right foot forward. Position the hand just slightly above the shoulders. Now position your body so that you are a foot and a half in front of your hand.

FIGURE 2 As you lean forward, place your left hand on your thigh for balance. Next, as you lean forward, twist your left shoulder to the left and drop downward. As you do, you will begin to feel your chest and shoulders tighten.

SHOULDER STRETCH

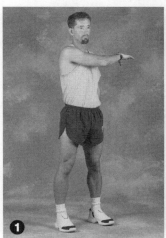 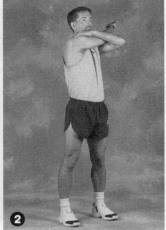

FIGURE 1 Bring your right arm across your chest. Wrap your left arm around the right elbow, placing your right elbow in the joint of the left arm.

FIGURE 2 As you do, place your left hand on your right shoulder. Squeeze your right arm against your chest. After 5 seconds of squeezing your arm against your chest, slowly elevate your right arm. Once finished, repeat to the opposite side, remembering to squeeze that arm against your chest and slightly pull it away from the shoulder.

TRICEP STRETCH

The key to this stretch is to maintain your back straight as you lean to one side or the other. If you twist your upper torso in any manner, you will take away from the effectiveness of this stretch. In other words, you will only rotate from one side to the other, not front and back.

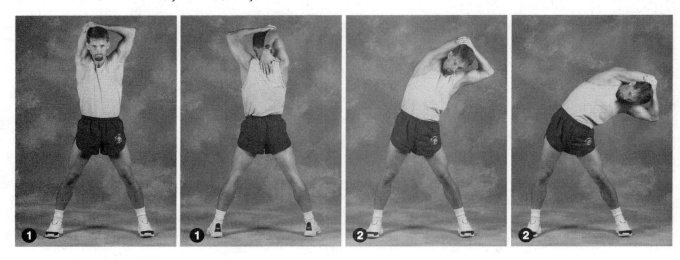

Figure 1 Place your right hand down the center/middle of your back.
Next, grab your right elbow with your left hand.

Figure 2 With your left hand on your right elbow, lean to the left. Once you have completed this, repeat with the opposite side. **Key Note**—maintain a downward press on the elbow as you lean.

PARTNER CHEST STRETCH

This is a slow and methodical stretch. But this does not mean that when your partner says good that you let his or her arms fling like rubber bands. Release your partner's wrists slowly.

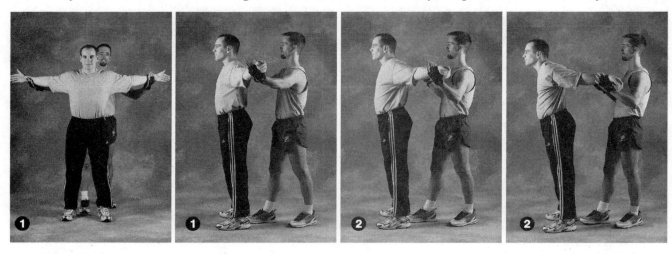

FIGURE 1 Place your hands straight out at your side with the thumbs up and palms facing forward.

FIGURE 2 Your partner grabs your wrists and begins to slowly pull them back toward each other. Once you have reached the point of discomfort, stop and hold it for 5 seconds. Next, slowly let your hands return to the original position. During this movement keep their arms at or just below shoulder height.

ARM ROTATIONS

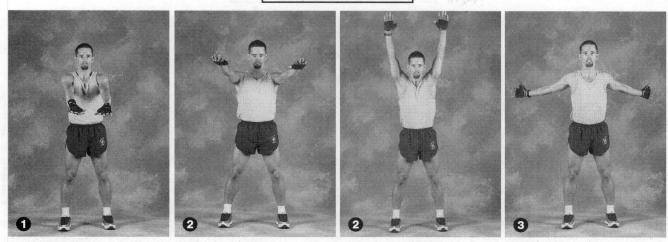

FIGURE 1 Put your arms out in front at waist height with feet spread shoulder-width apart.

FIGURE 2 Begin to rotate arms up and back. Bring your arm as close to the ears as possible during this rotation.

FIGURE 3 Repeat stretch but in a forward motion.

MID EXERCISE STRETCHES

The following stretches will be performed while performing various upper and lower body exercises.

COBRA STRETCHES

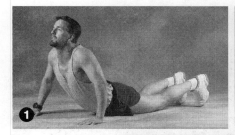 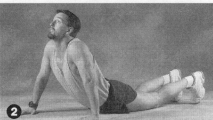 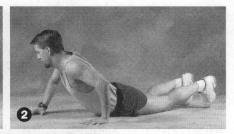

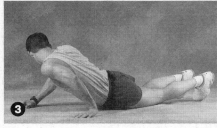 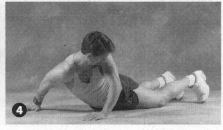

FIGURE 1 Lie flat on the ground with your hips placed firmly against the ground.

FIGURE 2 Lift your upper body to the point that your arms lock. Next, shrug your shoulder toward your ears.

FIGURE 3 Drop your left shoulder and pull your upper body to the right. This is similar to the tricep stretch but while in the prone position.

FIGURE 4 Repeat Figure 3 but to the opposite side.

UP, BACKS, AND OVERS

The key to this stretch is when you reach upward, extend your arms outward and back, forming a wide V. The same motion will be performed as you bring your arms back. You want to feel the tightness in your chest and shoulders.

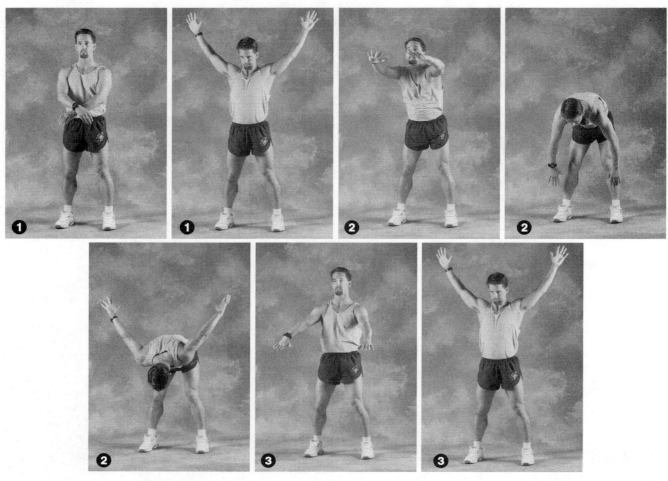

FIGURE 1 Lift your arms straight up and over your head. As you do, tilt your upper torso back a little. Open your arms out as you go back. Go past your shoulders.

FIGURE 2 Bring your arms back down and rotate them back so that they are behind your shoulders. Push this position to the point that your deltoids are tight.

FIGURE 3 Now rotate your arms in a complete 360° circle.

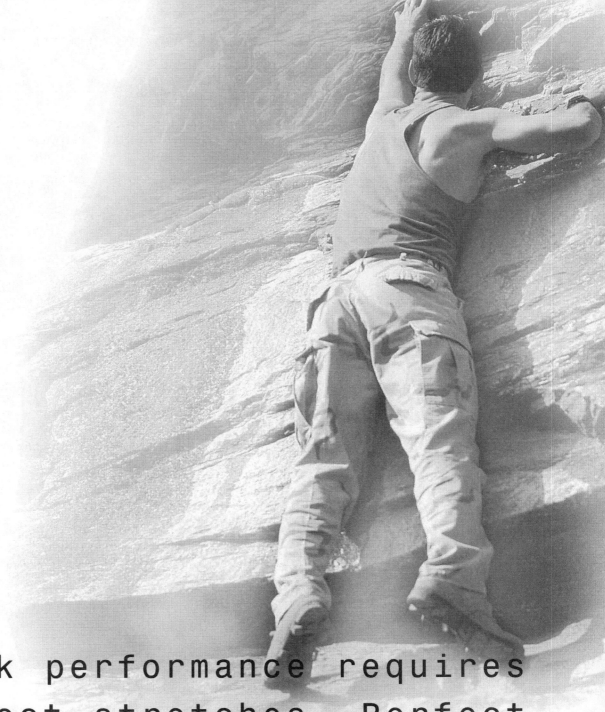

Peak performance requires
perfect stretches. Perfect
stretches require time.

PERFORMANCE

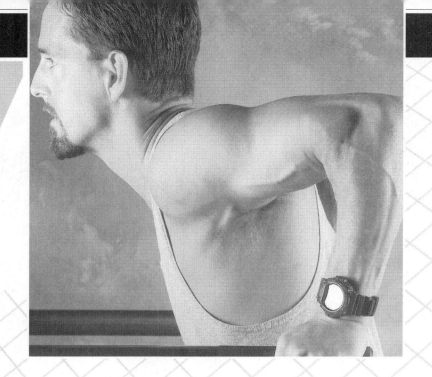

7

The key to functional strengt
is perfect technique.

UPPER BODY EXERCISES

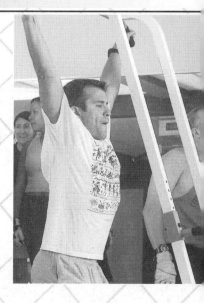

Upper body—what an interesting topic. Most people think that if they go to the gym, hit the bench hard, and develop a well-defined chest, then they have reached their goal. The fact remains that the chest is just a small step in the development of a functional upper body. As a matter of fact, Americans in general have very neglected backs. So what we want to accomplish with the upper body section is to develop core strength, functional muscles that look good yet perform flawlessly. I cannot emphasize enough, technique, technique, technique. We want full range of motion in every exercise you perform.

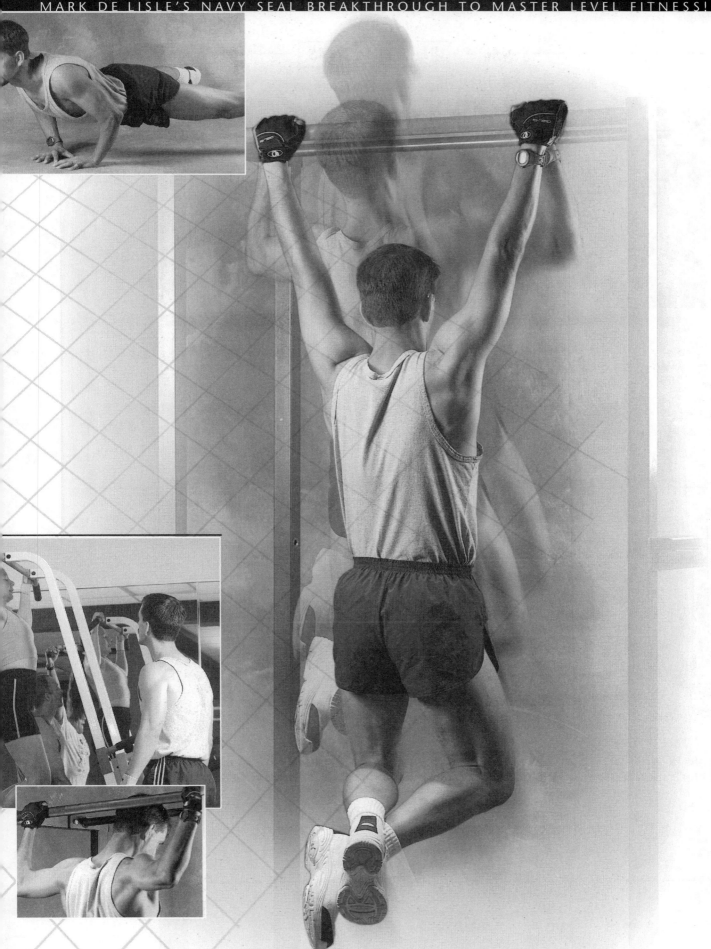

NECK ROTATIONS

This exercise will be performed in a counterclockwise motion. To get the most out of this exercise you need to perform the higher repetitions.

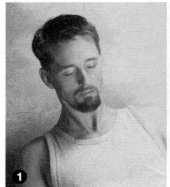 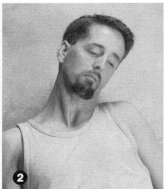 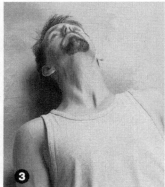 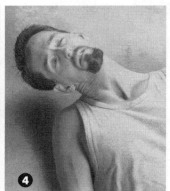

FIGURE 1 Lift your head straight up.

FIGURE 2 Rotate your neck counterclockwise to the side.

FIGURE 3 Continue rotating your head to the middle position.

FIGURE 4 Rotate your head to the right side.

While performing this exercise, you will utilize the four-count method.

(1-2-3-1) (1-2-3-2) (1-2-3-3)

BACK CONTRACTIONS

To get the most out of this exercise you need the higher repetitions.

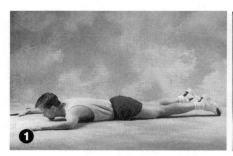 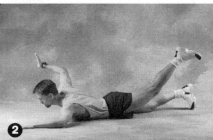 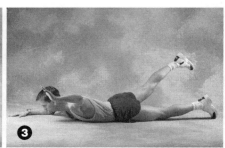

FIGURE 1 Lie on your stomach with your arms at a 90° bend to the side.

FIGURE 2 Simultaneously raise your right hand with your left foot.

FIGURE 3 Now raise your left hand in conjunction with your right foot.

The count will be performed in the following manner: (1-2-1) (1-2-2). As you lift your right hand and left foot, this is 1. As you lift your left hand and right foot, this will be 2. The final count on the repetition is when you bring all hands and feet back to the starting position.

SWIMMERS EXERCISE

This exercise is a combination of a reversed flutter kick and a swimmer's breaststroke.

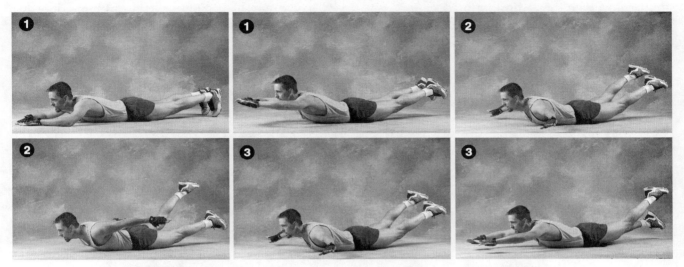

FIGURE 1 Lie on your stomach with your arms in front of you,
hands 4 inches off the ground and touching. Lift your feet 4 inches off the ground.

FIGURE 2 Start by raising your left foot first. Bring your hands down to your side while
maintaining them 2 inches off the ground until they hit your side. While doing so, lift your
right foot off the ground. Pretend to kick your feet as you would in the water.

FIGURE 3 As you perform this exercise, your feet will alternate positions,
one rising up after the other. Your hands during this process will be going from
above your head to your side, back and forth.

BACK LIFTS

It is very important to be very methodical about this exercise. This is not a speed exercise and
should be done in a slow and smooth fashion.

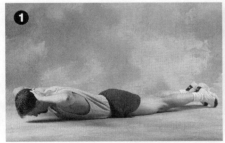 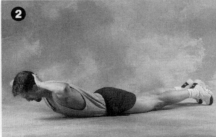 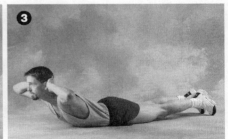

FIGURE 1 Lie on your stomach with your hands crossed behind your head.

FIGURE 2 Raise your head and upper torso off the floor at least 4-6 inches.

FIGURE 3 Lower your upper body back down in a smooth and slow manner.

REGULAR PULL-UPS

I have never found another exercise that works more interactive muscle groups than pull-ups. This one simple movement has a profound effect on your upper body, strength, endurance, and physique. It is an excellent exercise to strengthen your back, which is the most neglected body region of personal fitness. If you want maximum results, pay close attention to technique. It is very easy to break technique to ease out an extra rep. I would rather have you hang at a 90° bend in your elbow, giving all you have, than to have you cheat to raise your chin to the bar. I want to see full range of motion through these exercises. If you have a bend in your elbows at the end of your motion, your technique is wrong.

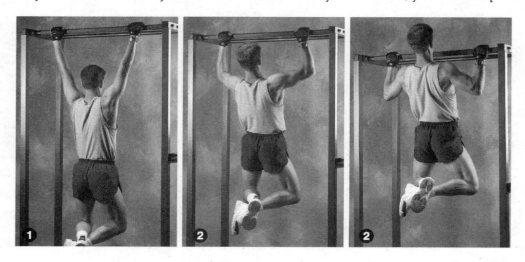

FIGURE 1 To find the right-hand position look up at the bar as you place your hand on it. Follow this position down to your shoulders. There should be a nice even V in your position. If your hands are straight above your shoulders, they are too close together.

FIGURE 2 Lead with your chest with your neck extended. Pull down with your elbows, utilizing all the muscles in your back.

The best advice I received in doing pull-ups was to block out everything around you. Visualize only the muscles that are used in this movement. This will allow you to actually focus more on technique and push out those extra reps that you desire.

I have never found another exercise that works more interactive muscle groups than pull-ups.

INTERACTIVE

CLOSE GRIP PULL-UPS

The key to making close grip pull-ups successful is the distance you give between your hands. If you are inexperienced with pull-ups, I recommend that you keep a good 2-inch separation between your hands. As you improve in technique, begin to close the gap to the point that your hands are touching each other.

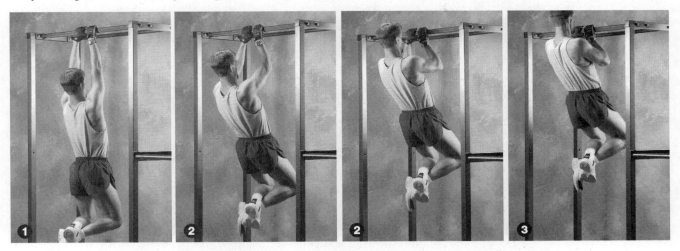

FIGURE 1 Start from a hanging position.

FIGURE 2 As you begin to elevate yourself, maintain an even distance between your elbows. Do not flair your elbows out.

FIGURE 3 Once your chin is level with the bar, begin to lower yourself to the original position.

REVERSE GRIP PULL-UPS

The same technique used with close grip pull-ups will be adapted in this exercise, with the following difference. Begin with a 3-inch separation in your hands, but do not close the gap past a 1-inch separation.

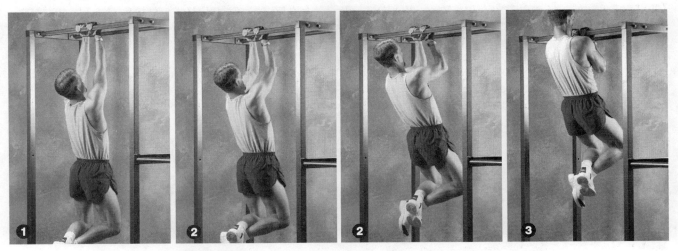

FIGURE 1 Once again start from a dead hang.

FIGURE 2 As you begin to elevate your body, lead with your chest. This allows you to focus on your bicep as you bring yourself into the bar.

FIGURE 3 Bring your chin up to the level of the bar and slowly lower yourself back down again.

BEHIND THE NECK PULL-UPS

This is a tremendous exercise for developing the back. Especially the inner back region. To get the most out of this exercise keep your head position up. Most enthusiasts have a tendency to drop their head in order to reach the back of their neck.

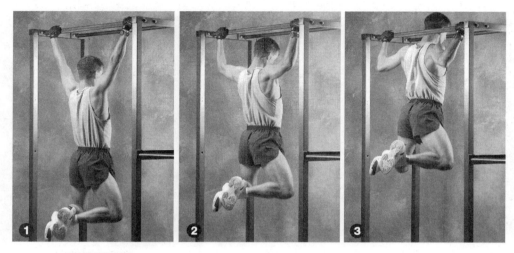

FIGURE 1 Take a slightly wider grip on this exercise.

FIGURE 2 Keep looking straight ahead as you reach the base of your neck.

FIGURE 3 Touch the base and slowly lower yourself back down.

Do not lean too far forward during this movement.
Your shoulders should rise up directly underneath the bar, not in front of it.

COMMANDO PULL-UPS

Commando is another great pull-up for the triceps, deltoids, and upper back.

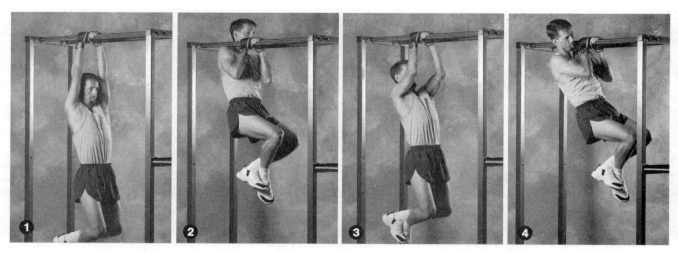

FIGURE 1 Left hand is placed directly in front of the right hand.

FIGURE 2 Begin elevating yourself to your right shoulder.

FIGURE 3 Lower yourself to the 45° angle or just past.

FIGURE 4 Raise yourself back up to your left shoulder and slowly return to the starting position.

WIDE ANGLE PULL-UPS

This movement will really open up your back. Wide angles are a tremendous pull-up for increasing size, especially around the shoulder blades.

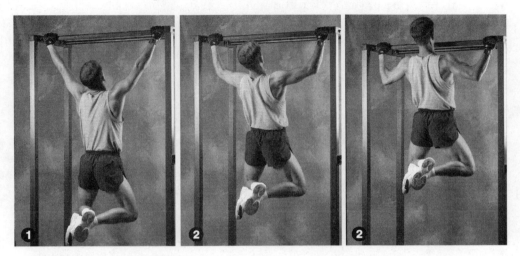

FIGURE 1 Extend your hands at least 6 inches past the shoulders.

FIGURE 2 Utilize the same movement that was used in regular pull-ups.

BAR DIPS

Having exhausted the back and shoulder muscles through pull-ups, dips help transition to the chest muscle. Dips work the shoulders, triceps, and chest. This way you can finish off the shoulders and prep the chest and triceps for push-ups. For this reason it is important to maintain the dips after the pull-ups and before the push-ups. You can modify the routine as you wish but keep in mind that the routine has been created in the format it is in for certain reasons.

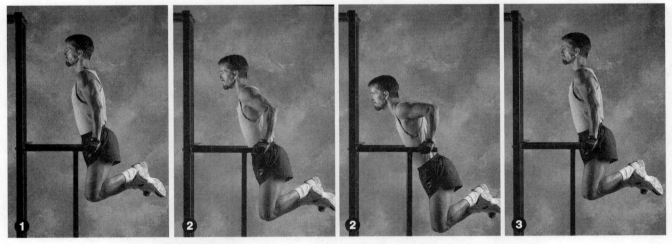

FIGURE 1 Keep your eyes focused straight ahead.

FIGURE 2 In a controlled fashion begin lowering yourself to a 90° bend. The biggest mistake I find is that most exercisers will only drop down about 2 inches.

FIGURE 3 Fully extend all the way back up. Helpful hint—keep your knees tucked or hanging directly underneath your hip.

REGULAR PUSH-UPS

The key to an effective push-up is the distance between the hands. Too many exercisers' hands are too close together. The perfect position for regulars is determined by the position of your forearm in the 90° bend stage. When your arms are in the 90° position, your forearms should be straight up and down. If your elbows are flaring out past your hands, then your hands are too close together. Also, watch your hip placement. Do not allow your back to bow or to have your rear too high in the air.

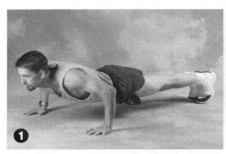 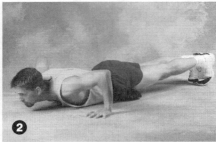 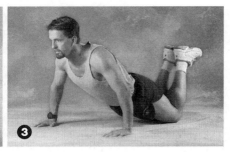

FIGURE 1 Proper hand position with your hands, back straight, feet together, head looking forward.

FIGURE 2 Drop down to your chest or worst case scenario 90° bend.

FIGURE 3 With any of the push-ups, if you are not able to perform them, I recommend you do them from your knees. Or if you tire out early, drop down to your knees. These exercises are too valuable to skip over.

DIAMOND PUSH-UPS

Diamonds are a great exercise for the triceps if done properly. Most mistakes are made when the diamond in your hand is placed under your shoulders. The diamond should be placed on the lower sternum.

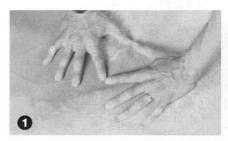 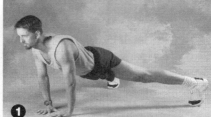 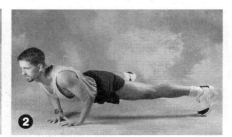

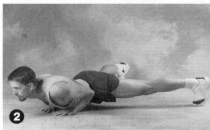 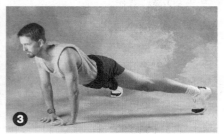

FIGURE 1 Make a diamond with your hands. Place your feet wider than shoulder-width apart.

FIGURE 2 Lower your body so that your hands touch your lower chest.

FIGURE 3 Return to starting position.

FIGURE 1 Spread your feet more than shoulder-width apart. The hands should be slightly wider than shoulder width. Now bring your hands within 2-3 feet from your feet.

FIGURE 2 Start to go down as if you were going under an imaginary fence. Your chest should begin to scrape the ground right around the palms of your hands. You could even scrape the ground 2 inches prior.

FIGURE 3 Go past your hands about 10 inches and begin to make your way back.

FIGURE 4 It now becomes a pushing motion, not a lifting. Push back toward the wall behind you and do not lift up. Your head should end up between your arms.

If you tire during this exercise, drop down to your knees after Figure 2 and continue on through the motions.

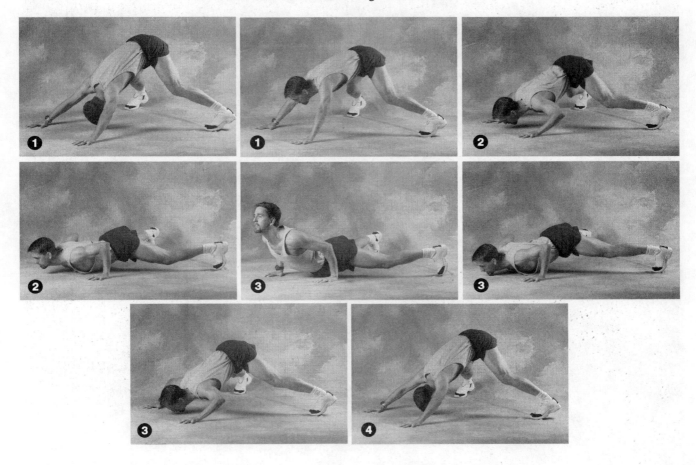

Compromise technique and you compromise results.

EIGHT COUNT BODY BUILDERS

This exercise is excellent to get the heart pumping and to finish off your push-up routine. It can also be used as a warm-up exercise but keep the repetitions low.

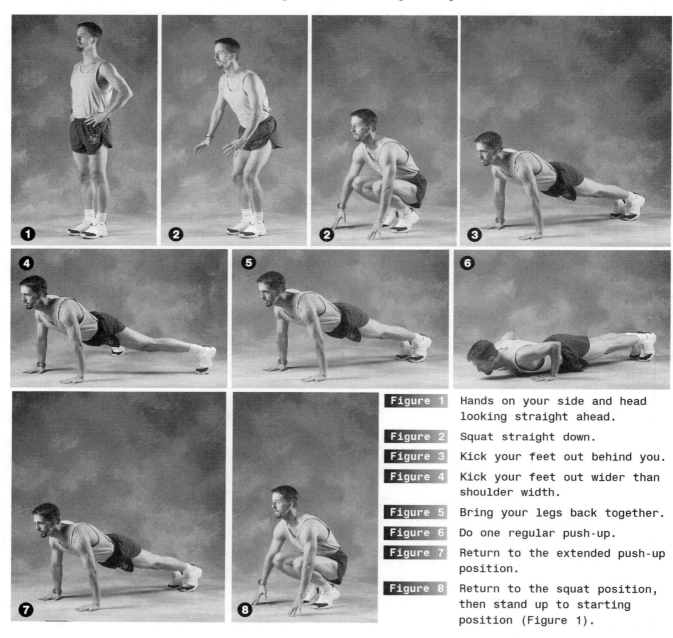

Figure 1	Hands on your side and head looking straight ahead.
Figure 2	Squat straight down.
Figure 3	Kick your feet out behind you.
Figure 4	Kick your feet out wider than shoulder width.
Figure 5	Bring your legs back together.
Figure 6	Do one regular push-up.
Figure 7	Return to the extended push-up position.
Figure 8	Return to the squat position, then stand up to starting position (Figure 1).

Do the same amount of exercises in 10 percent less time. It forces your muscles to work harder and improves your endurance.

ENDURANCE

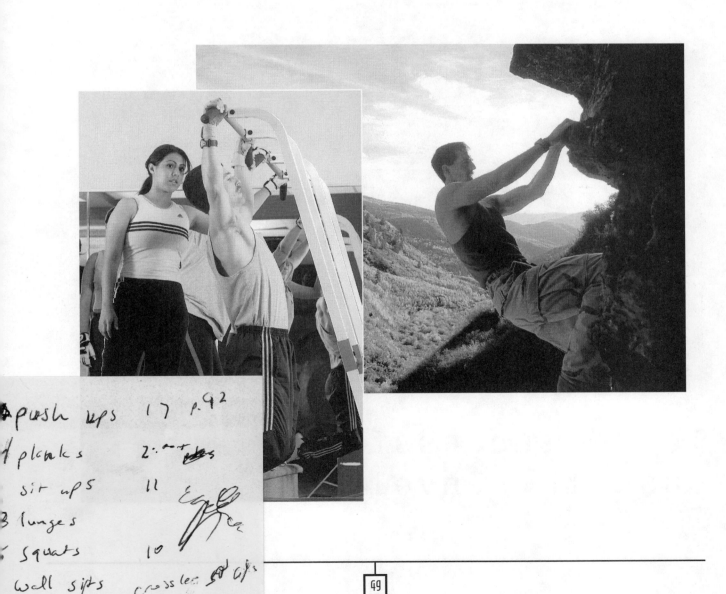

push ups   17 p.92

planks   2: ...

sit ups   11

lunges

squats   10

wall sits   crosslec
            squat jumps

MODIFICATION EXERCISES

To be successful in any exercise routine, you must push the envelope. Make yourself get out of its comfort zone. Modification will allow you to do so whether you are exercising for the first time or you have peaked out. Modifications will allow you to keep going.

MODIFIED PUSH-UPS

Maybe you have never done push-ups before, but you know the benefits are great. By starting from your knees, you can work up to standard push-ups. The only problem is that many people use modifications as a crutch. Modifications are to be used as an assistance. I always want you to try to use a regular position first every time. When you have pyramided and there is nothing left, this is the time when you would drop to your knees and perform the modified position. At this time you drop to your knees, which will allow you to push out a couple more reps. You will experience tremendous gain by utilizing this method.

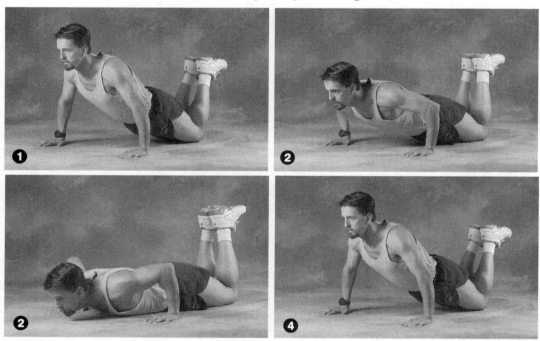

FIGURE 1 Start from your knees with your hands in the proper position, back straight, and your legs raised at a 45° bend. Keep your feet together and your head looking forward.

FIGURE 2 Drop down to your chest or worst case scenario 90° bend.

FIGURE 3 Return to the starting position.

To be successful, you must push the envelope.

MODIFIED DIAMOND PUSH-UPS

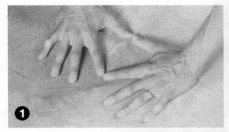
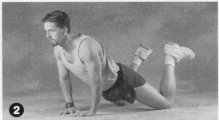
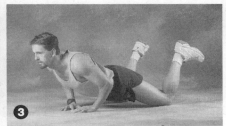

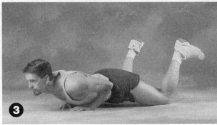
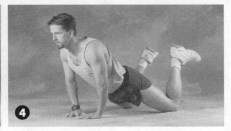

FIGURE 1 Make a diamond with your hands.

FIGURE 2 Start from your knees with your hands in the proper position, back straight, and your legs raised at a 45° bend. Keep your head looking forward.

FIGURE 3 Drop down to your chest or worst case scenario 90° bend.

FIGURE 4 Return to the starting position.

MODIFIED DIVE BOMBERS

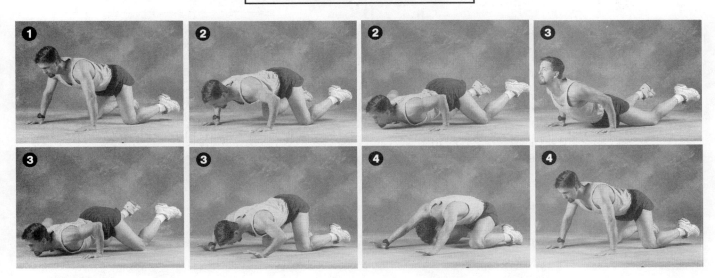

FIGURE 1 Start from your knees. The hands should be slightly wider than shoulder width. Now bring your hands within 2-3 feet from your feet.

FIGURE 2 Start to go down as if you were going under an imaginary fence. Your chest should begin to scrape the ground right around the palms of your hands. You could even scrape the ground 2 inches prior.

FIGURE 3 Go past your hands about 10 inches and begin to make your way back.

FIGURE 4 It now becomes a pushing motion, not a lifting. Push back toward the wall behind you and do not lift up. Your head should end up between your arms. Return to starting position.

MODIFIED PULL-UPS

Same reasoning behind modifications for pull-ups. Use your thigh muscles to assist in the lift. Do not use this method as an escape goat. This modification is only to assist.

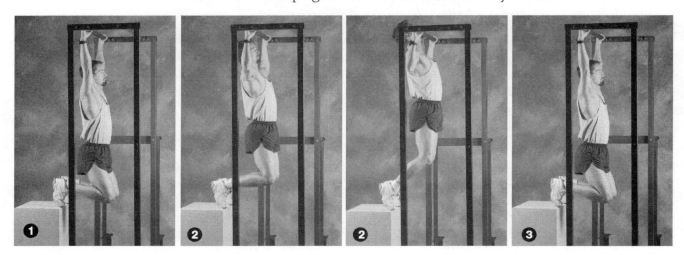

FIGURE 1 Place your feet on a chair, stool, or platform. It is important to use the balls of your feet and toes for maintaining position and pushing. If you place your upper feet in the down position, then you will not be stable.

FIGURE 2 Use just your thighs and feet for lifting yourself.

FIGURE 3 Return to the starting position.

MODIFIED DIPS

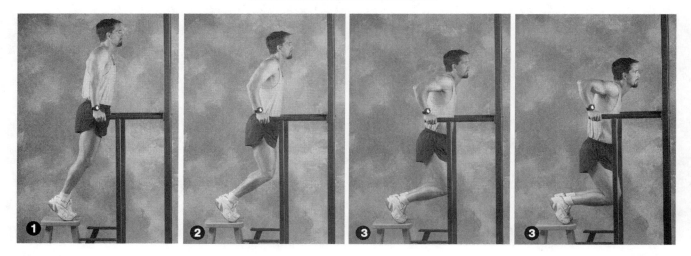

FIGURE 1 Place your feet on a chair, stool, or platform. It is important to use the balls of your feet and toes for maintaining position and pushing. If you place your upper feet in the down position, then you will not be stable.

FIGURE 2 Use just your thighs and feet for lifting yourself.

FIGURE 3 In a controlled fashion begin lowering yourself to a 90° bend. The biggest mistake I find is that most exercisers will only drop down about 2 inches. Return to the starting position.

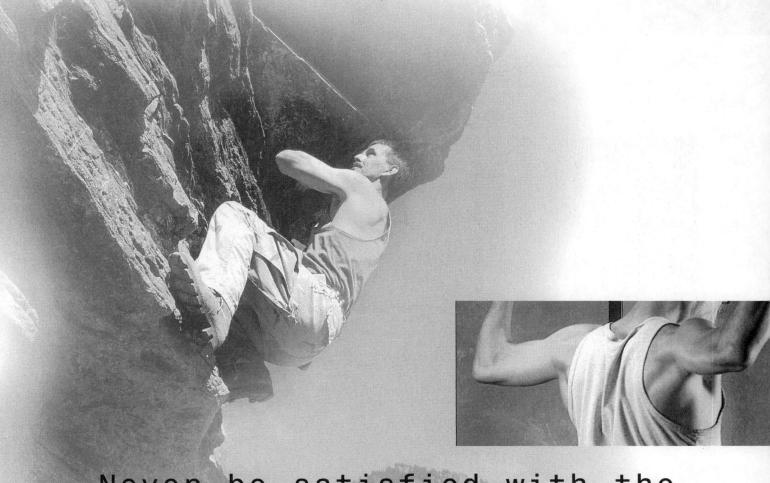

Never be satisfied with the fitness level you are working on—until you reach your final goal. Continually push yourself to go past your limits. Only when you push yourself will you be capable of achieving the results and fitness level you desire.

SATISFIED

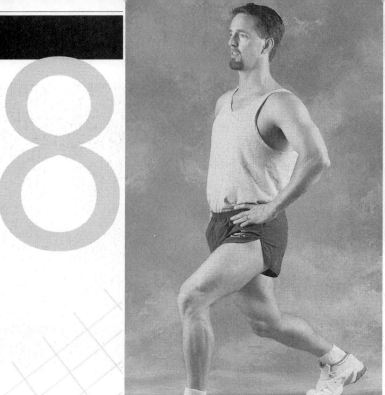
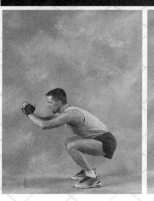
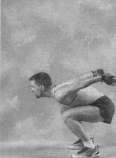

LOWER BODY EXERCISES

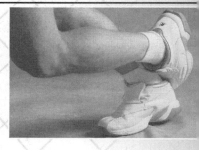

This section on leg exercises has been the most requested in this greatly anticipated sequel to *Navy SEAL Exercises*. I have been kicking myself for some time now for omitting this part from the original manual. The good part is that we have developed some very effective routines since then and look forward to your reaction to this new section.

The same principle applies to this section as in the other sections. You must keep the rest periods short to maintain the burn you are looking for and to receive cardio benefits from the exercises.

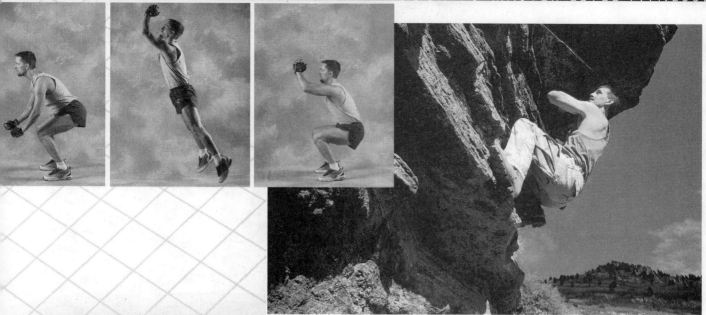

Maintain the burn.

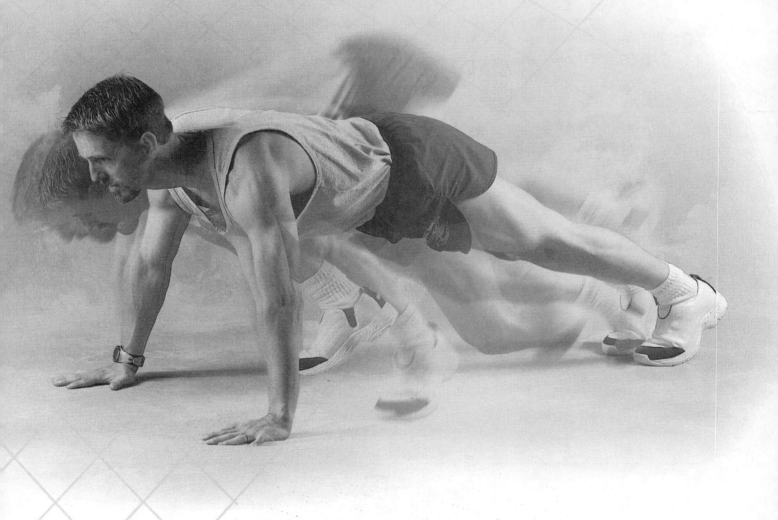

LUNGES

Be slow and methodical on this exercise. Technique must be the most important objective here so you do not damage your knees. If you have tender joints, do not drop your knees all the way to the ground but rather drop down two inches, then three, and so on. As you begin to strengthen the joints, you may be able to push yourself a little harder. But it is always better to suck up the ego and play it safe. Why push it and end up hurting yourself. You not only stop your progress, but it may take weeks for recovery.

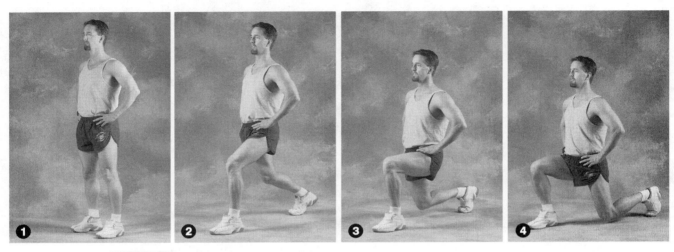

FIGURE 1 Stand with your feet together and your hands on your hips.
FIGURE 2 Step forward with your left leg to the point that you have 3-3½ feet between your feet.
FIGURE 3 Lower your right knee to the ground and create a 90° bend in the left leg. Once again place your right arm or forearm on the thigh of your right leg.
FIGURE 4 Repeat the process with your left leg.

The key here is to lower the opposite knee to the ground so that it barely touches the surface while maintaining a 90° bend in the other leg. You may have to extend your initiating foot out a little farther to get the exact effect you want.

It's always better to suck up your ego and play it safe.

SQUATS

As simple as this exercise may seem, if done with the higher repetitions it can be very effective. But it should not be your first exercise. You need to exhaust the thighs and hamstrings through lunges first.

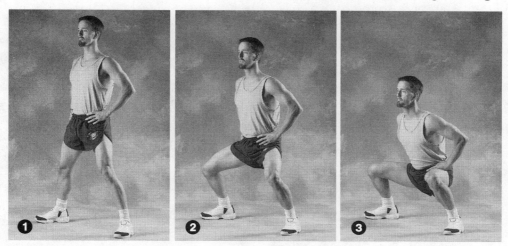

Figure 1 Legs should be spread more than shoulder-width apart with hands on your hips. Have the tips of your toes pointing outward slightly. By doing so your shoulders will not lean forward. You may also want to hold your arms straight out in front of you.

Figure 2 The key to this exercise is to lower your hips as you maintain your lower back straight and just drop your buttocks directly down to a 90° bend. Look straight ahead, chest forward. DO NOT LOWER YOUR SHOULDERS FORWARD AND HUNCH YOUR BACK!

Figure 3 As you raise yourself back to the original position, squeeze your buttocks and drive with your legs.

THE WALL

That's right, "The Wall"—no explanation for this one. Plain and simple, it stinks, it's a pain, and it hurts. None of this 30-second stuff either.

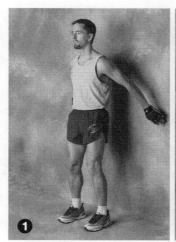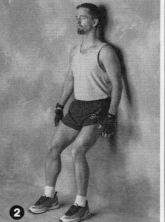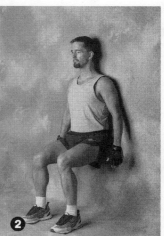

Figure 1 Place your back flat against the wall with your legs shoulder-width apart.

Figure 2 Slowly lower yourself down to a 90° bend in your legs. No hands on the thighs or hips, and for the last 10 seconds of this exercise I want you to push as hard as you can against the wall. Feel the burn!

STAR HOPS

There is no getting around the fact that if you do this one in public, people are going to look at you funny. No worry, just tell them the SEALs do them! As ridiculous as you may look performing this exercise, you are going to feel it too!

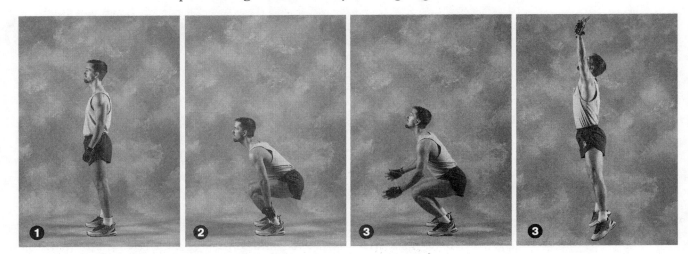

Figure 1 Legs shoulder-width apart and arms naturally down at your sides.

Figure 2 Squat straight down as if you were performing regular squats. Reach down and touch your ankles.

Figure 3 Explode up into the air as hard as you can. As you attempt this, extend your arms and legs outward as demonstrated in the photo.

Return to the original position. There are no rest periods between reps.

Star Hops and Frog Hops are great exercises for the fast twist muscle. The key to these is to perform this exercise various times with only a 15-second rest period in between each set.

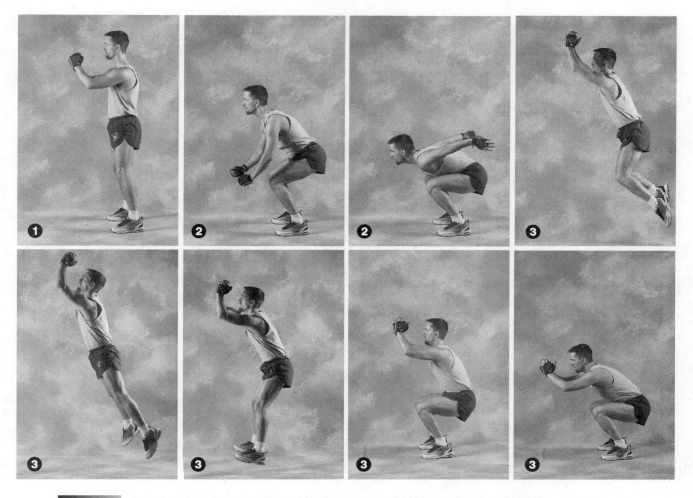

Figure 1 Stand straight up with your hands at chest level, feet shoulder-width apart.

Figure 2 Squat down as you prepare to thrust forward with everything you have. The key to this motion is arm position. Start with your arms at a 90° bend behind you.

Figure 3 Thrust forward while maintaining your squat position. Use the momentum of your arms thrusting forward to help you extend your distance. Do not land stiff-legged. Think of your legs as a shock absorber. If the shocks on your car do not retract all the way back up, your ride would be very rough. In Frog Hops, as you land let the force bring your legs back down slightly past the 90° bend. Far too many exercisers land without bending their legs. Land with the heels first, and as you rock forward, rotate to your toes while bringing your arms back again. Once in the original position, launch again.

FIRE HYDRANTS

This is another one of those exercises that is not the most masculine looking,
but it is extremely effective.

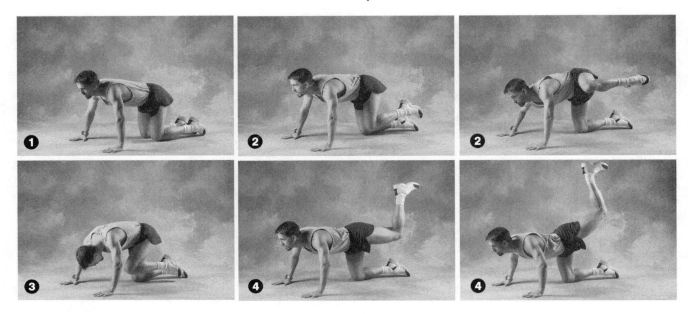

Figure 1   Hands on the ground with your knees directly under your hips.
Figure 2   Lift your left leg directly out to the side.
Bring it straight back to the original position.
Figure 3   Bring your left knee toward your chest as you contract your abs at end.
Figure 4   Raise your left foot straight up but do so flat-footed right
up toward the ceiling. If you raise your foot up at an angle, you are wrong.
Make sure you lead with the heel.
It must rise straight up as if following a pole right up to the top.

Switch sides and repeat.

This exercise is meant to give you a cardio boost along with burning the leg muscles. Don't be surprised if you feel the burn in your arms too.

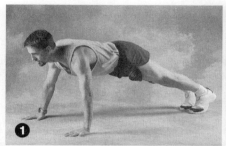 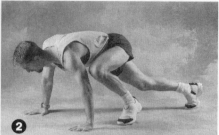

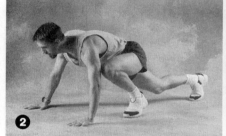 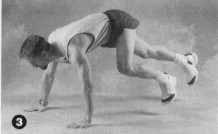 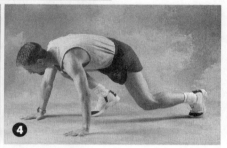

Figure 1 Put yourself in the push-up position.

Figure 2 Bring your left knee to your left elbow.

Figure 3 Bring your left knee back to the starting position.

Figure 4 Bring your right knee to your right elbow and return it to the starting position.

"Pain is weakness leaving the body."
—An old SEAL saying.

CALF LIFTS

As simple as this exercise looks, when you get into the higher repetitions it will burn. Be careful to not overdo it on these. Recently, I pushed it really hard in a workout and literally could not walk the following day. I looked as though I had been riding bareback on a horse for a week. This exercise can work, and do not be alarmed if you feel the burn in the arches of your feet. This is natural, and as you become conditioned to this exercise, your feet will adjust.

STRAIGHT FOOTED

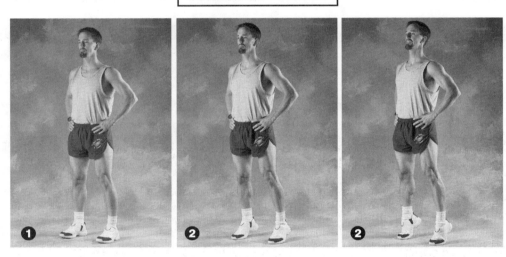

Figure 1 Feet shoulder-width apart and hands on your hips.

Figure 2 Lift your entire body up until you are fully extended on the balls of your feet. Contract the calf muscle for half a second and go back down. At full extension there should be at least a 2- to 3-inch separation from the heel to the floor.

TOE TO TOE

Your feet will have a tendency to open back up while performing this exercise.
Go ahead and adjust them back to the original position throughout the exercise.

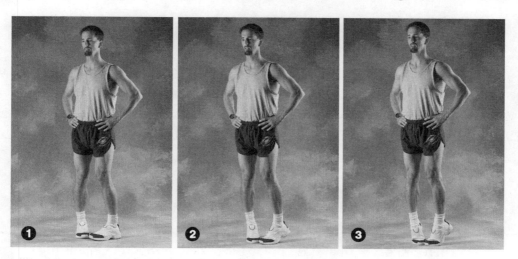

Figure 1 Point toes inward so that they touch and place your hands on your hips.

Figure 2 Lift your entire body up until you are fully extended on the balls of your feet.

HEEL TO HEEL

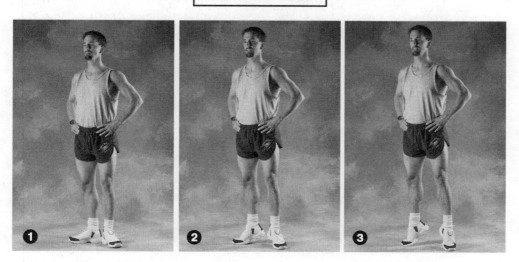

Figure 1 Heel to heel with at least a 6-inch gap in between
the front part of your toes. Hands on your hips.

Figure 2 Lift your entire body up until you are fully extended on the balls of your feet.

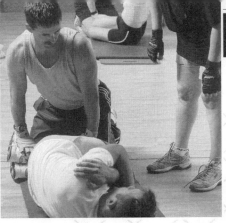

9

ABDOMINALS

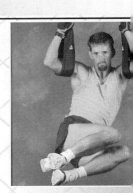

Abs are one of the most neglected parts of your body. To get the most out of your ab routine you need to keep the repetitions high and rest periods in between short. An ab routine will always be effective if you maintain proper form and technique.

There are many opinions on what is correct form and what is not, and which exercises are proper and which are not. Every routine can be criticized either for effectiveness or improper exercises. The main priority is to take as much stress off the lower back as possible. But if you go too easy you won't see any results to your abs and back. The point is to move at a safe and moderate pace. As you progress, you will find that some exercises that normally would have been just for the advanced can now be yours. Which brings us right back to starting with realistic goals and desires and working toward them.

Pace yourself through your routine. Only do the exercises that you feel you are safe to do at this stage of your conditioning. As you get stronger, add one exercise to your routine that would be considered advanced. Keep the repetitions low on this exercise as compared to the rest of your routine. Every two weeks add one more exercise after another. Before you know it, you will be completing the entire routine at an advanced level.

As you perform the lower abdominal exercises, you will notice that your body has a tendency to raise the lower back, especially with exercises such as the Flutter Kicks and Knee Roll Ups. To help keep proper form, if you raise your head and shoulder blades off the mat while performing the proper technique, your lower back will stay flat on the mat. As soon as you lay your head down from fatigue, your lower back will begin to arch. Technique, not the numbers, is the key here.

Technique,
perseverance,
goals, and
desire will get
you there.

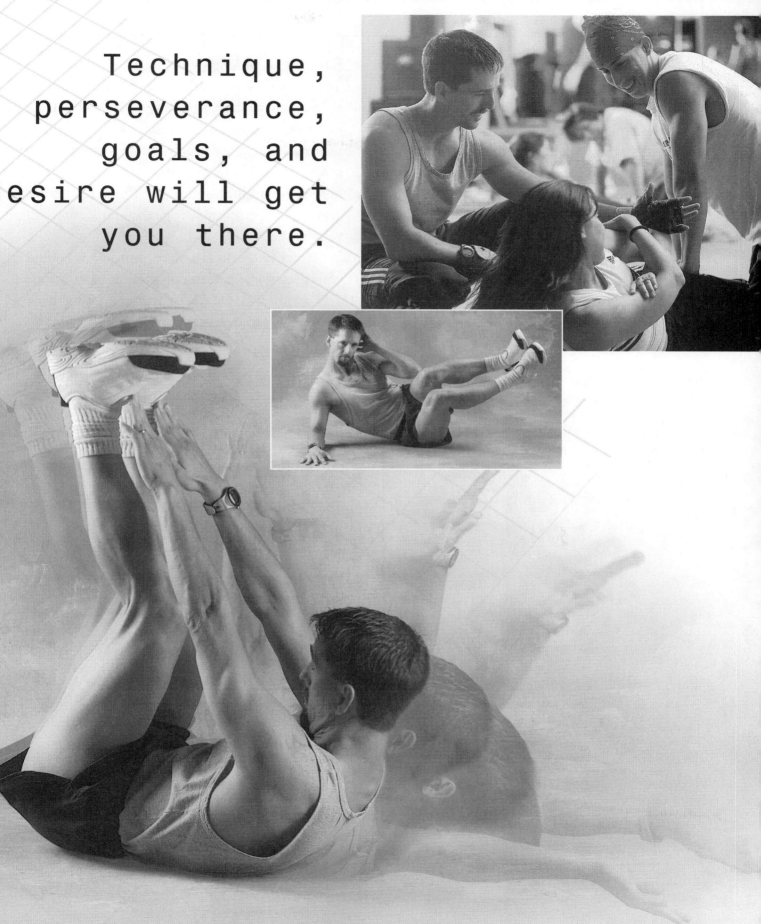

Your abs are going to burn, and you are going to feel as though you cannot do any more, but you are wrong. Your mind is giving up on you and wanting to cop out. Push past the fatigue and make yourself do the extra reps. You are not going to die; you are going to get tough. Remember an old SEAL saying: "Pain is weakness leaving the body." Again, do not keep going if you feel a sharp pain. There is a distinction between fatigue and pain.

If you have sweated, pushed hard, done everything the book has said, and yet gain no six pack, it is usually because you have a layer of excess baggage sitting around your stomach. You can have the strongest abs in the world and no one will ever know unless you burn the calories to make them show. You have to burn that layer off before your stomach muscles will show. Take the time to include a good running, swimming, or cardio program into your fitness routine. The goal here is overall fitness, not just a rock hard body. Technique, perseverance, goals, and desire will get you there.

Please note: Do not place your hands behind your neck while performing abdominal exercises. This action will add excess pressure on the neck and could lead to injury.

X SIT-UPS

The starting position for this exercise is lying flat on your back. Each time you touch an elbow to your knee, you must return to this original position. This is not a speed exercise, and you actually get better results when you slow this one down. The crucial part to this exercise is that you must lift your shoulder blades off the ground. As you cross over from one side to the next, do not relax your abs and lower your shoulders back down. You must keep them elevated and abs tight as you rotate from side to side.

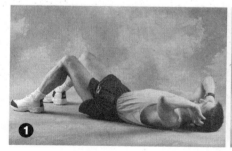 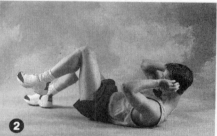 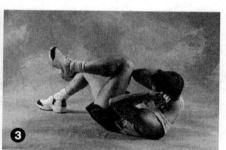

Figure 1 On your back, **hands on your ears.** Legs bent, feet shoulder-width apart.

Figure 2 Bring your left knee so that it is centered just above your belly button.

Figure 3 At the same time crunch your right elbow to the same position so that the two touch.

Lower your right elbow and left knee back down to the original position. Then begin with the right knee and the left elbow.

The counting for this exercise goes as followed: 1-2-1, 1-2-2, 1-2-3, and so on.

You will notice that the shoulder blades never relax during this entire movement.

Maintain your foot at knee level or above on the leg that is moving toward the elbow. Don't let your feet drop lower than your knee when your elbow is touching the knee.

This is one of my favorites. When I do high enough repetitions with this one, I always get a good burn.

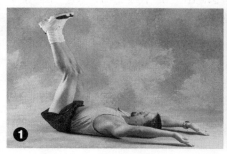 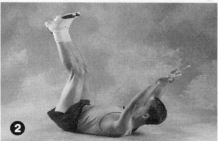 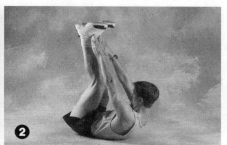

Figure 1 Hands above your head and feet at a 75°-90° bend.
Legs slightly bent at the knee.

Figure 2 Reach as high as you can and try to touch your feet or at least your ankles.
Slowly bring yourself back down to the original position.

CRUNCHES

Crunches have been around for a long time, but they are still a great exercise. The most common mistake made with this exercise regards the position of the legs. Many people have a tendency to bring their knees past the 90° position, so that their knees are closer to their elbows. What will make or break the effectiveness of this exercise is to keep your abs tight through the entire movement. Stay with the proper position, and you'll be pleased with the results. Be sure to maintain your feet at knee height.

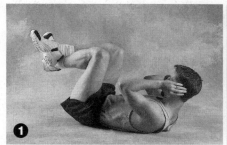 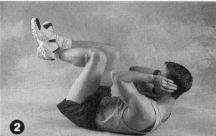 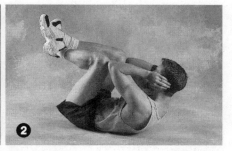

Figure 1 Hands on your ears. Feet up in the air with a 90° bend in your legs. Do not drop your feet below your knees.

Figure 2 Raise your upper torso toward your thighs by leading with your elbows.
You want a direct line from your elbows to your lower thigh muscles.
Return to the starting position.

Many fitness enthusiasts will tighten their abs while raising their upper torso, but as soon as they touch their shoulder blades they relax. As they are ready to perform the next repetition, they actually jerk their upper torso into beginning the motion. Wrong! Take this movement nice and slow and do not let the tension off until you are finished with the set.

SIDE SIT-UPS

This remains a very effective exercise if done correctly. A common mistake occurs when people twist their upper torso and do not lift both shoulder blades off the floor. From the photos, imagine having a string attached to your elbow and connecting with your upper knee. If you are not following this pattern, the movement is wrong. There is no twisting involved. You are raising your left shoulder blade toward your right knee. This movement will cause your right shoulder blade to rise just slightly off the floor. Another tip is to place your opposite hand on your obliques to feel the movement.

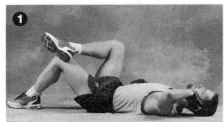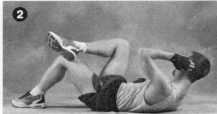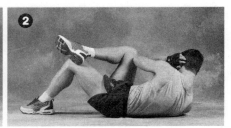

Figure 1 Place your right foot over your left knee and your left hand by your left ear.

Figure 2 Touch your left elbow to your right knee or lower thigh.

Figure 3 Return to the original position and switch legs.

OBLIQUES

This is another exercise I have repeated from the first book because of its effectiveness. There are a few key techniques that make or break this exercise. It is a common mistake to bring your knees toward your chest as you perform this exercise. At no point during this exercise should you move the knees except in an up and down motion. Another common mistake is to not bend your upper torso toward your thigh as your knees rise off the ground. As you observe the photos, key on the fact that I am crunching my obliques to get the most out of it. Note also the method in which you are to raise your legs. Pretend as though someone has attached a piece of string to your ankles. Now the difference, raise your feet and knees together at the same level with the feet slightly above the knees.

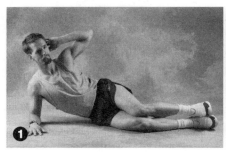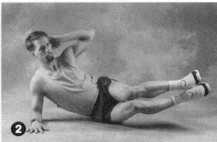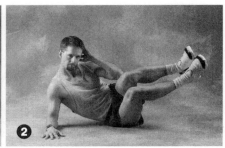

Figure 1 Lie down on your right side. Prop yourself up on your right elbow. Left hand placed by your left ear.

Figure 2 Raise your feet and legs together. Your legs should have just a slight bend to them.

Figure 3 As your feet and leg reach 12-18 inches off the ground, begin to extend your left elbow toward the side of your middle thigh.

Slowly return to the original position.

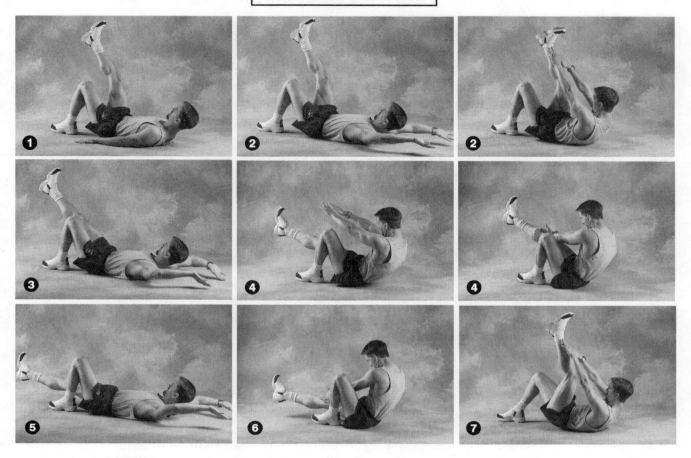

Figure 1 Raise your right foot so that it is at least 3 inches above
your left knee or to 90°.

Figure 2 Hands above your head, reach and touch as high as you can.
For some it may be your toes; for others it may be your shins.

Figure 3 Now without lowering your foot, rest for 5 seconds. Lower your right
foot to a 45° position. This should be around the level of your left knee.

Figure 4 Hands above your head, reach and touch as high as you can.
In this position try to touch your shin. At the minimum, touch your knee.

Figure 5 After resting for 5 seconds, lower your right foot to about 6 inches off the floor.

Figure 6 Hands above your head, at least touch your knees.
If you are just starting out, touch your thighs.

Figure 7 Rest 15 seconds and switch legs. Don't panic!
By changing legs you actually can keep going despite how you feel.

This is a great exercise if you are short on time.

PARTNER SIDE SIT-UP

This is a difficult exercise and should only be performed after you have reached a level of comfort with the other Side Sit-ups. The key to making this exercise effective is to maintain your partner's lower legs as stable as possible. As you face your partner who is performing the exercise, place your hands just below their knees. Place most of your pressure right underneath the knee and support the ankles without crushing their legs. You are only there to maintain support and allow their legs to be stable while they perform the exercise.

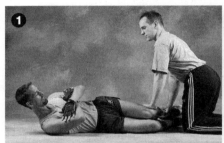 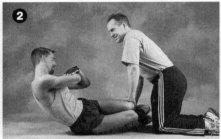 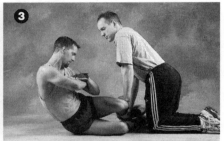

Figure 1 Lie down on your right side. Rotate your upper hip slightly outward. Cross your arms across the chest. Place a slight bend in your knees.

Figure 2 Have your partner face you as he or she places their knees right below yours. Have your partner apply pressure right underneath the knee while placing the right hand on the ankle or foot.

Figure 3 Begin to raise your upper torso so that at least your shoulders are off the ground. Your goal is to raise them to the point where you can touch your left elbow to your right thigh.

Return slowly to the original position and switch sides.

If you exhale forcefully at the top of the movement, you'll force your abs to work harder.

EXHALE

This is a more advanced exercise, and I recommend that you feel comfortable with the rest of the ab routines before trying this exercise. This is a slow and methodical movement. Anything else would be considered jerking your body into position, which can cause injury and defeats the purpose.

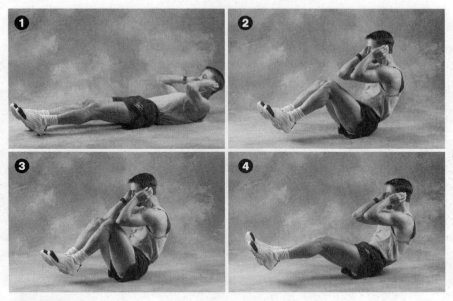

Figure 1 Lie flat on your back with your hands by your ears.

Figure 2 As you simultaneously raise your legs and upper body to meet, bend your knees as if to do a sit-up.

Figure 3 Crunch your ab muscles as your elbows touch your lower thighs or knees.

Figure 4 As you slowly lower yourself back down, begin to straighten your legs out again. Just as your shoulder blades are about to touch, repeat the exercise. Your feet never rest on the ground during this entire exercise.

FLUTTER KICKS

Flutter Kicks are a fun exercise that are good for the lower back, lower abs, hip flexors, etc. What makes this exercise effective is the correct position of the head. Many exercisers try to perform this exercise with their heads flat on the floor, but when they lift their legs their lower back begins to arch. Obviously, this is not what we want. So even if you are tired, do not lower your head to the floor as you perform the repetitions. If you have to, it is better to lower your feet so they rest on the ground rather than lower your head. While performing this exercise, you want a slight bend in your legs, but not so much that it looks as though you are riding a bicycle. We do not bend our legs that much!

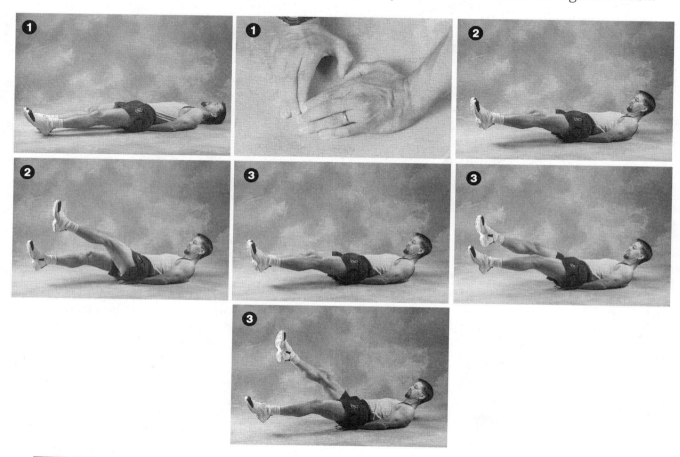

Figure 1 Lie flat on your back with your hands underneath your lower hips or buttocks.

Figure 2 Lift your head and begin to raise your left leg from 6-36 inches. At no time are you to let your feet rest on the ground.

Figure 3 As your left leg returns to the 6-inch position, begin to raise your right leg to the same 36-inch position.

Return your right leg to the original position and begin again with the left leg. Your counting will go as follows: 1-2-3-1, 1-2-3-2, 1-2-3-3, 1-2-3-4

This is an advanced exercise, but it can be achieved by anyone at any age. I have two 62-year-old grandmothers in my exercise class who perform this exercise routinely. However, I do not recommend doing this exercise until you are in really good shape. Always consult your doctor before performing any advanced exercise routine.

It is very important that your partner use control and not throw your legs back down too hard. But if your partner does not exert enough momentum in the throw down, then you will not get the full effect from this. The object of the exercise is to grab your partner's ankles and raise your feet up to his or her chest. Then they throw your feet down toward the ground, hard enough to make it difficult for you to stop them before they hit the ground. To make this exercise fun, your partner needs to perform this exercise in a pattern, and then after so many reps begin to throw the feet down in broken patterns. For example, once to the left, then to the right, then to the middle, next back to the right, next to the left, and next to the middle. This way the exerciser never knows which way the feet will go, and he or she will have to maintain their ab muscles tight the entire time. So begin with 3 to the middle, 3 to the right, and 3 to the left. Afterward you can begin breaking up the pattern.

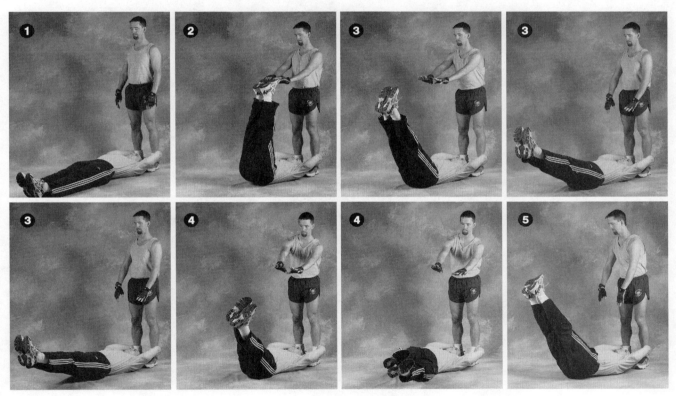

Figure 1 Lie on your back as your partner places their feet right at the base of your head.

Figure 2 Grab your partner's ankles as you raise your feet to their chest.

Figure 3 Partner——throw the feet down to the middle three times in a row. Once again, smoothly!

Figure 4 Just as the exerciser's feet reach your chest again, throw the feet down to the left.

Figure 5 Next, throw your partner's feet down to the right twice in a row.

For a set period of time begin to throw their feet down in an irregular pattern.

Return to the original position.

REVERSE CRUNCHES

Reverse Crunches are a great way to work your lower abs. Keep your abs tight during the entire movement of this exercise. Once you place yourself into proper position, do not move your legs. Lock that position in your legs and maintain it during the entire movement.

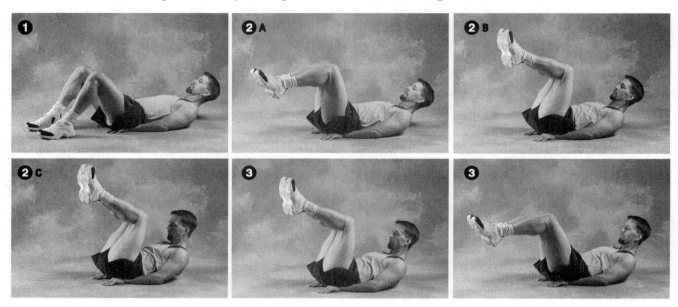

Figure 1 Lie flat on your back with your head raised up. Place your hands underneath your hips.

Figure 2 Maintain your legs in a reversed V position. Raise legs toward your chest to the point that your knees are just past the 90° position.

Important: you will notice in the 2C that I crunch into my knees as the legs break the 90° bend. This will greatly enhance the exercise.

Figure 3 Return your legs to the original position while maintaining the V position. To keep your lower back flat on the deck, keep your head elevated during the entire movement.

To get the most out of this movement, as you roll your knees to your chest kick your feet up toward the ceiling at the end by at least 2 inches. Do not roll your legs up toward your chest so much that your lower back breaks a 90° angle.

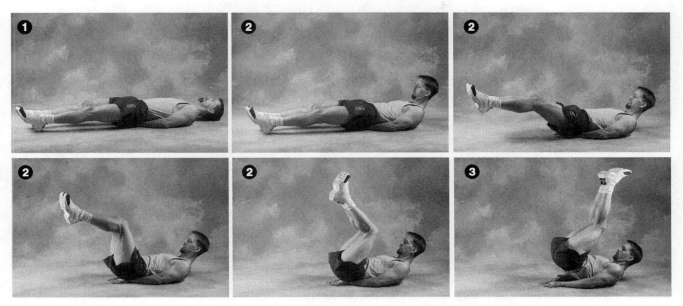

Figure 1 Lie flat on your back with your hands underneath your lower hips.

Figure 2 Begin to raise your feet off the ground and bring your knees to your chest.

Figure 3 Lift your feet toward the ceiling so that your lower back rises up off the ground by at least 2 inches. Slowly lower your feet back down and return to the starting position.

You can work your invisible abdominal muscles and flatten your waistline when you suck in your gut.

ABDOMINAL

AB BANDS

Ab Bands are a great way to take pressure off the lower back and still get a terrific abdominal work-out. At the same time, they are a good way to finish off your routine. There are many exercises that can be done with the Ab Bands, but in this book we are going to concentrate on two.

FULL RANGE HANGING LEG RAISES

What makes this exercise most effective is to raise your knees to your chest with the feet extended past the knees. Many people tuck their feet under their knees as they raise their legs. You will receive so much more from this movement if you just lower your feet out in front of your knees and keep them out in front the entire sequence.

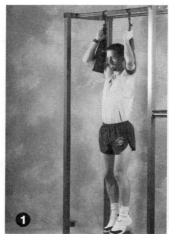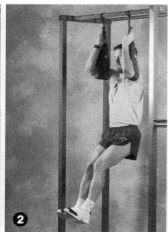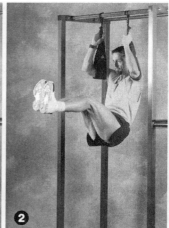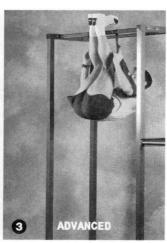

Figure 1 Tuck the bands under your armpits to the point that they are snug under your arms. The key is to be comfortable.

Figure 2 Slowly raise your legs to your chest or as close as you can. As you reach the peak of the movement, you should tighten your abs the best you can.

Slowly lower your legs . . . very slowly.

Figure 3 This movement is extremely advanced and should only be used after conquering all other levels.

You will definitely feel a good burn on these, especially at the end of your workout. If you have a partner, a helpful tool is to place your partner's hand off to the side. Place your partner's hand just high enough so that you have to fully lift your heels to hit the palm of the hand. When you have a target to aim for, it helps improve performance and technique.

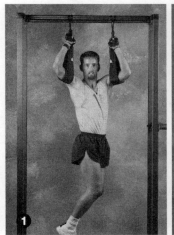 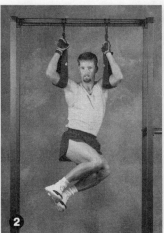 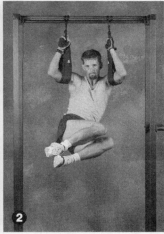 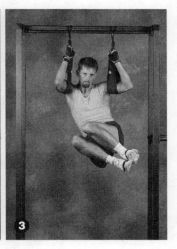

Figure 1 Set yourself comfortably in your bands. Once you are comfortable, rotate your hips to the side.

Figure 2 Similar to obliques, lift your legs and heels at the same time and crunch into your sides. Try to lead with your feet.

Figure 3 Reverse sides once you have finished required amount of reps. Slowly lower your legs down to the starting position.

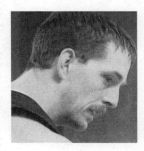

" You will definitely feel a good burn. "

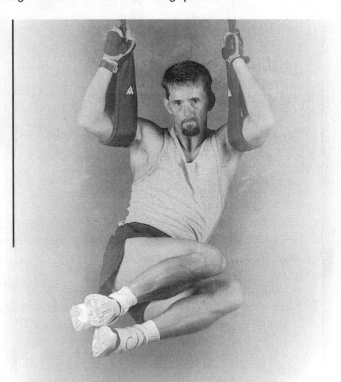

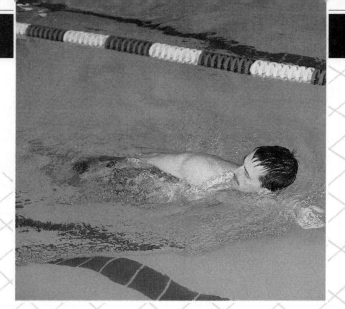

10

ROUTINES

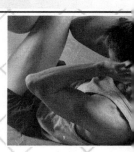

My best advice for establishing workout routines is to learn to listen to your body. As you become more and more in tune with your body and muscle groups, you will begin to know what is effective and what is not, what your limits are and when you can push a little more. Keep adjusting each routine to better meet your goals.

I recommend that you first utilize the routine as stated below in the three days a week format, then as you grow and become more aware of yourself, begin to adjust it. After six years of working with various body types and various fitness levels, I have found that you do not need to work out five days a weeks *if you are doing upper body along with lower body all in one shot.* As an alternative, you work out five days a week by doing upper body one day and lower body the next. Anything beyond that and you are pushing your body too hard. The key to growth is your rest period.

If you are weightlifting, you need to give your muscle groups a much longer rest period. But with calisthenics you do not need to. So stick to the three times a week, and you will be just fine. If you do not have time to run or swim on the same day, it might be a good idea to do so on your off days.

The key to
growth is your
rest period.

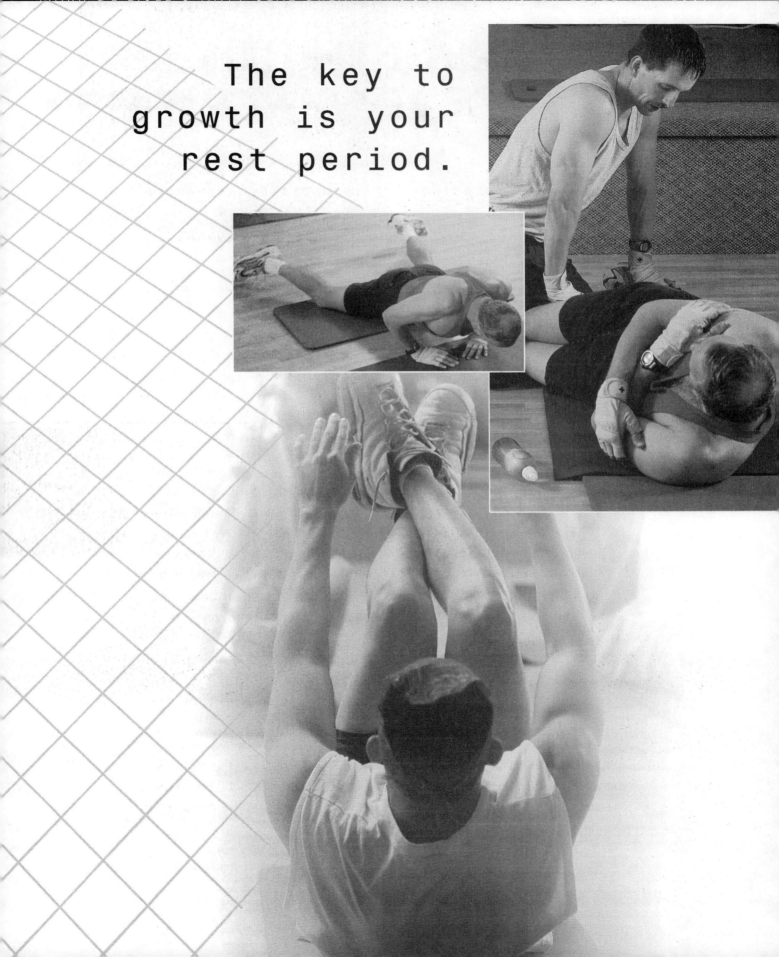

MONDAY EXERCISE ROUTINES

	SUNDAY	MONDAY	TUESDAY	WEDNESDAY	THURSDAY	FRIDAY	SATURDAY
Legs & Abs							

WARM-UPS	BEGINNING	INTERMEDIATE	ADVANCED
Jumping Jacks	25	35	45
Running in Place	30 seconds	60 seconds	60 seconds
Half Jumping Jacks	25	35	45

STRETCHES

Bend Overs
Cross Overs
Inner Thigh Stretch
Forward Lunge Stretch
Side and Oblique Stretch
Hurdler Stretch
Butterfly
ITB Stretch
Sitting Thigh Stretch
Calf Stretch

LEGS			
Lunges	10 (2 count)	35 (2 count)	45 (2 count)
Squats	20	45	60
Fire Hydrants	10 (each side)	25 (each side)	40 (each side)
Mountain Climbers	10 (4 count)	20 (4 count)	30 (4 count)
The Wall	1 minute	2 minutes	3 minutes
Calf Raises			
Straight Footed	50	75	100
Toe to Toe	50	75	100
Heel to Heel	50	75	100

ABS	90°/45°/6"	90°/45°/6"	90°/45°/6"
Clockwork Sit-ups	15 / 10 / 5	25 / 20 / 15	50 / 45 / 40
Hand to Toes	10	25	50
X Sit-ups	10 (2 count)	25 (2 count)	50 (2 count)
Crunches	10	25	50
Side Sit-ups	10	25	50
Obliques	10	25	50
Atomics		20	40
Knee Bends	10	25	50
Flutter Kicks	10 (4 count)	25 (4 count)	50 (4 count)
Reverse Crunches	10	25	50
Chest Roll-ups	10	25	50

TUESDAY EXERCISE ROUTINES

Upper Body

STRETCHES	BEGINNING	INTERMEDIATE	ADVANCED
Chest Stretch			
Lat Stretch			
Shoulder Stretch			
Tricep Stretch			
Partner Chest Stretch			
Arm Rotations			

UPPER BODY WORKOUT

	BEGINNING	INTERMEDIATE	ADVANCED
Neck Rotations	10 (4 count)	20 (4 count)	40 (4 count)
Back Contractions	10 (2 count)	20 (2 count)	40 (2 count)
Swimmer Exercise	10 (2 count)	20 (2 count)	40 (2 count)
Back Lifts	10	15	20
Regular Pull-ups	2-4-2	2-4-6-8-10-8-6-4-2	8-10-12-14-12-10-8
Close Grip Pull-ups	1-2-1	2-4-6-8-6-4-2	6-8-10-12-10-8-6
Reverse Grip Pull-ups	1-2-1	2-4-6-8-6-4-2	6-8-10-12-10-8-6
Commando Pull-ups	1-1-1	2-4-6-4-2	4-6-8-6-4
Behind the Neck Pull-ups	1-2-1	2-4-6-4-2	4-6-8-6-4
Bar Dips	5 (4 sets)	10 (4 sets)	20 (4 sets)
Regular Push-ups	2-4-6-8-6-4-2	2-4-6-8-10-12-10-8-6-4-2	10-12-14-16-18-20-22-24-22-20-18-16-14-12-10
Diamond Push-ups	2-4-6-4-2	2-4-6-8-10-8-6-4-2	8-10-12-10-8
Dive Bombers	2-4-6-4-2	2-4-6-8-10-8-6-4-2	8-10-12-10-8
8 Count Body Builders	5	10	20

WEDNESDAY EXERCISE ROUTINES

	SUNDAY	MONDAY	TUESDAY	WEDNESDAY	THURSDAY	FRIDAY	SATURDAY
Cardio Day							

WARM-UPS	BEGINNING	INTERMEDIATE	ADVANCED
Running in Place	30 seconds	45 seconds	60 seconds
Jumping Jacks	30	45	60
Half Jumping Jacks	30	45	60

CARDIO	BEGINNING	INTERMEDIATE	ADVANCED
Walking Lunges*	20 yards (2 times)	30 yards (3 times)	40 yards (4 times)
Running in Place**	20 yards (2 times)	30 yards (3 times)	40 yards (4 times)
Frog Hops	20 yards (2 times)	30 yards (3 times)	40 yards (4 times)
Star Hops	10	15	20
Mountain Climbers	10 (4 count)	15 (4 count)	25 (4 count)
Sprints (look to appropriate sections)			

*1 repetition means up and back

**Running in Place in this section is actually High Knees.
As you jog the 20/30/40 yards, pump your knees up and down as fast as you can.

ABS			
Full Ranging Hanging Leg Raises	10	30	45
Hanging Side Raises	10 (each side)	30 (each side)	45 (each side)
Short Contractions			
Hand to Toes	10	30	45
Crunches	10	30	45
Side Sit-ups	10	30	45
Obliques	10	30	45

THURSDAY EXERCISE ROUTINES

Upper Body

WARM-UPS	BEGINNING	INTERMEDIATE	ADVANCED
Running in Place	30 seconds	45 seconds	60 seconds
Jumping Jacks	30	45	60
Half Jumping Jacks	30	45	60

STRETCHES

Chest Stretch
Lat Stretch
Shoulder Stretch
Tricep Stretch
Partner Chest Stretch
Arm Rotations

UPPER BODY WORKOUT

	BEGINNING	INTERMEDIATE	ADVANCED
Neck Rotations	10 (4 count)	20 (4 count)	40 (4 count)
Back Contractions	10 (2 count)	20 (2 count)	40 (2 count)
Swimmer Exercise	10 (2 count)	20 (2 count)	40 (2 count)
Back Lifts	10	15	20
Regular Pull-ups	2-4-2	2-4-6-8-10-8-6-4-2	8-10-12-14-12-10-8
Close Grip Pull-ups	1-2-1	2-4-6-8-6-4-2	6-8-10-12-10-8-6
Reverse Grip Pull-ups	1-2-1	2-4-6-8-6-4-2	6-8-10-12-10-8-6
Commando Pull-ups	1-1-1	2-4-6-4-2	4-6-8-6-4
Behind the Neck Pull-ups	1-2-1	2-4-6-4-2	4-6-8-6-4
Bar Dips	5 (4 sets)	10 (4 sets)	20 (4 sets)
Regular Push-ups	2-4-6-8-6-4-2	2-4-6-8-10-12-10-8-6-4-2	10-12-14-16-18-20-22-24-22-20-18-16-14-12-10
Diamond Push-ups	2-4-6-4-2	2-4-6-8-10-8-6-4-2	8-10-12-10-8
Dive Bombers	2-4-6-4-2	2-4-6-8-10-8-6-4-2	8-10-12-10-8
8 Count Body Builders	5	10	20

FRIDAY EXERCISE ROUTINES

Legs & Abs

	SUNDAY	MONDAY	TUESDAY	WEDNESDAY	THURSDAY	FRIDAY	SATURDAY

WARM-UPS	BEGINNING	INTERMEDIATE	ADVANCED
Jumping Jacks	25	35	45
Running in Place	30 seconds	60 seconds	60 seconds
Half Jumping Jacks	25	35	45

STRETCHES
Bend Overs
Cross Overs
Inner Thigh Stretch
Forward Lunge Stretch
Side and Oblique Stretch
Hurdler Stretch
Butterfly
ITB Stretch
Sitting Thigh Stretch
Calf Stretch

LEGS			
Lunges	10 (2 count)	35 (2 count)	45 (2 count)
Squats	20	45	60
Fire Hydrants	10 (each side)	25 (each side)	40 (each side)
Mountain Climbers	10 (4 count)	20 (4 count)	30 (4 count)
The Wall	1 minute	2 minutes	3 minutes
Calf Raises			
Straight Footed	50	75	100
Toe to Toe	50	75	100
Heel to Heel	50	75	100

ABS	90°/45°/6"	90°/45°/6"	90°/45°/6"
Clockwork Sit-ups	15 / 10 / 5	25 / 20 / 15	50 / 45 / 40
Hand to Toes	10	25	50
X Sit-ups	10 (2 count)	25 (2 count)	50 (2 count)
Crunches	10	25	50
Side Sit-ups	10	25	50
Obliques	10	25	50
Atomics		20	40
Knee Bends	10	25	50
Flutter Kicks	10 (4 count)	25 (4 count)	50 (4 count)
Reverse Crunches	10	25	50
Chest Roll-ups	10	25	50

WEEKLY ROUTINE BREAKDOWN

SUNDAY	MONDAY	TUESDAY	WEDNESDAY	THURSDAY	FRIDAY	SATURDAY

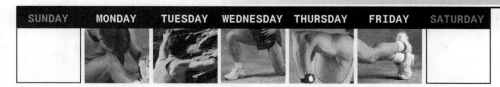

WEEK 2

Monday—Regular Legs/Abs

Tuesday—Regular Upper Body

Wednesday—Regular Cardio/Abs

Thursday—Circuit Training

Friday—1 Minute Interval Leg Workout/Abs

WEEK 3

Monday—Burnout with Legs/Abs

- Start out with 3 minutes on The Wall
- Next, hit lunges, squats, etc. to the point of exhaustion

Tuesday—Regular Upper Body

Wednesday—Regular Cardio/Abs

Thursday—Burnouts

Friday—Regular Leg Workout/Abs

WEEK 4

Monday—Regular Leg Workout/Abs

Tuesday—Contraction Workout

Wednesday—Reverse Cardio Workout in Exercise Layout

Thursday—Regular Upper Body

Friday—Contraction Leg Workout/Abs

For more detailed workouts, refer to the workout workbook.

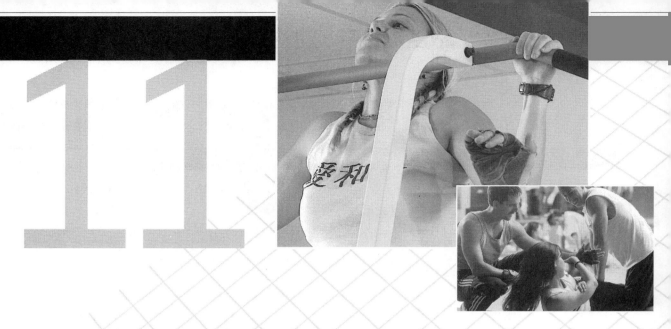

11

You are going to experience phenomenal gains in strength and endurance.

THE PYRAMID SYSTEM AND BLITZING ROUTINE

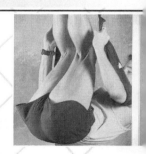

The pyramid system is what makes this entire program effective. The genius of the program, and the reason it works so much better than most exercise programs, is that it allows a person to not only peak once but multiple times during one exercise set. In a conventional program, for instance, you take a pull-up exercise and break it up into four sets of 10. During the first or second set, you probably will reach your peak with good form. To get through the last 2 sets, you must then compromise form to reach your 10, if you are pushing yourself hard through each set.

By way of contrast, let's say that 8 pull-ups is your peak. What makes the pyramid set so much more effective is that it takes you from 2 repetitions to 4 to 6 to 8. Your body will only peak once at its highest level, and if you try to peak again at the same level during your current set you are going to be disappointed. But by backing down the peak of the pyramid, you follow your peak of 8 with 6 to 4 to 2. The beauty is that you will experience the burning sensation of a peak all the way down the pyramid set. This is where you are going to experience phenomenal gains in strength and endurance.

A common question that follows is: "How long should I rest between each of my sets?" By way of example, for pull-ups I recommend that you perform 4 repetitions, drop off the bar, rest 15-30 seconds, then perform your 6. Once you have completed a full round on your pyramid set (2-4-6-8-6-4-2), then give your body a 60-90 second rest. Between sets, give yourself just enough time to recharge your body for the next exercise but not enough to let it cool down—that is the key. You will also be amazed that by changing the variation on your grip from one exercise to the next that you will be able to perform a completely new round of sets.

BLITZING ROUTINE

Blitzing is a routine specifically designed for the body to maintain peak burn. It is incredible for getting desired results quickly. This is particularly true when performing abdominal exercises, where it is very difficult to reach maximum burn by doing small numbers of reps. Also, by hitting a muscle group from multiple angles, you can guarantee that all facets of the group are being worked extensively. But like any other routine, the results will vary according to how you apply the rules.

The purpose is to systematically work from one muscle group to the next. For example, start with the upper abs, then move to your obliques, next to your middle abs, and last to your lower abs. This does not mean you cannot start with the lower abs and work your way up. I even recommend completely mixing up the entire ab routine on occasion, which does not mean that the blitzing routine is ineffective. Changing the routine shocks your body and helps to keep you from reaching one of those dreaded plateaus.

There are two key factors to getting the most out of your blitzing routine for the abs. First, very little time is given for the ab muscles to relax. By keeping your rest periods to 15-30 seconds, you do not allow the body to cool down. Second, focus on the contraction of your abdominal muscles. Time and time again I see exercise enthusiasts relaxing the ab muscles *during* the repetition. If you relax the abs, you will probably have to thrust your upper torso in a jerking motion to get back into motion once you have completed a movement. But if you keep your abs tight and contracted from start to finish, you actually double the results of this exercise. This is why I recommend that you raise your head off the floor and even try to maintain your shoulder blades off the floor. The payback is significant and fast!

Keep in mind that with small modifications in your technique, any exercise can take on a whole new meaning. I hear the comment all the time, "It's amazing how changing my position or maintaining contraction here and there changes the difficulty of the exercise." So lift your head off the floor, raise your shoulder blades, and keep your abs tight throughout the entire movement. By doing so, the blitzing routine will take on a whole new meaning, and your rest periods will be anxiously required.

12

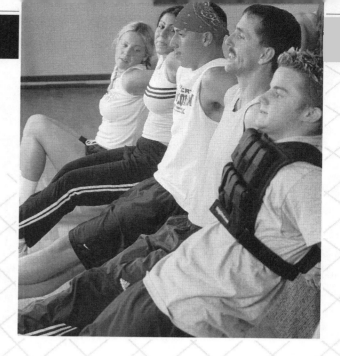

You can only get desired
results by plain old hard
work and sweat.

THE 15-MINUTE BLITZING ROUTINE

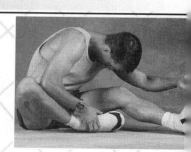

If you only have a few minutes to work out every day or just need to burn off some energy, I have picked my top exercises that you can combine together to get an incredible workout in just a short period of time. Obviously, you will not receive the same results or gains as you would if you applied the entire routine. There is no quick fix, and you can only get desired results by plain old hard work and sweat.

The key to any blitzing routine is your rest period in between each exercise. This does not mean that it is all sprint and no technique. As soon as technique goes out the window, injury and pain follow. Stick to the principles taught in the book and you will be fine. I would like to reinforce again that anyone attempting to exercise should consult a doctor before beginning, even if that means bringing the book to his office for approval.

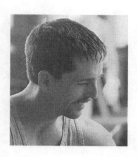

" The key to any blitzing routine is your rest period in between each exercise. "

Do each exercise to exhaustion. Except on abs and legs.

ABS

Hand to Toes	1:00 minute
Obliques	1:00 minute
Crunches	1:00 minute
Clockworks	1:30 total/45 sec per side
Full Range Hanging Legs	15 sec per position

PULL-UPS

Regular

Reverse Grip

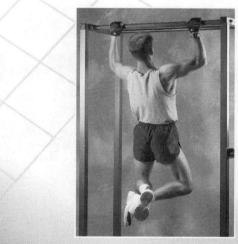

BAR DIPS

PUSH-UPS

Regular

Diamond

LEGS   1:30 EACH

Lunges

Squats

Regular Calf Raises

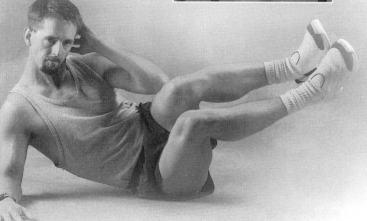

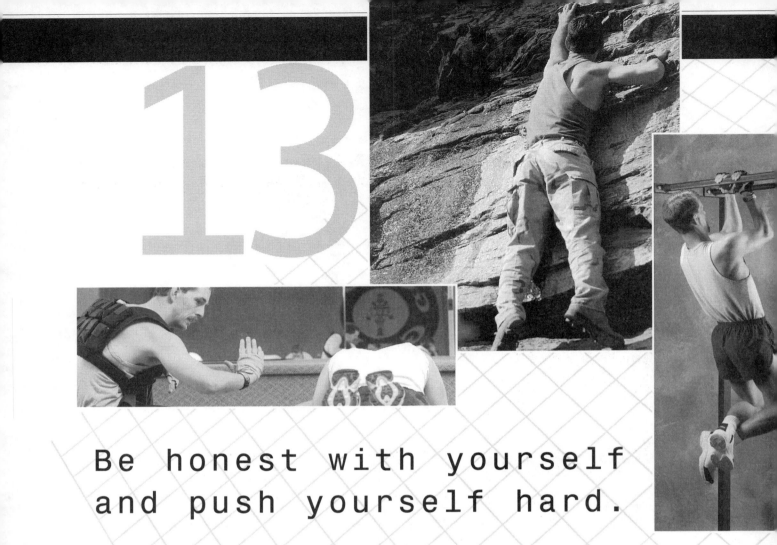

13

Be honest with yourself and push yourself hard.

NO, YOU ARE NOT READY FOR THIS!

Every routine needs a plateau breaker. The purpose of incorporating burnout routines into your workouts is to help shock the body and mess up its rhythm. This next part is very simple to follow, but it will be one of the toughest workouts you will ever encounter. You will be pushing yourself to your limits in one section and then be expected to go on to the next section and apply the same amount of effort. If you are not flat on your back with nothing left after this section, you are not pushing yourself hard enough.

Take this routine slowly and work yourself up to the levels you desire. Throw repetitions out the door and focus solely on your technique. There is no beginning, intermediate, or advance routines because it is based solely on your effort and output. Be honest with yourself and push yourself hard.

BURNOUT ROUTINE

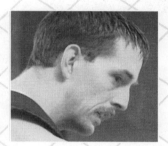

" You will be pushing yourself to your limits in one section and then be expected to go on to the next section and apply the same amount of effort. "

As many as you can do of each exercise.

STEP 1

Regular Pull-ups
Bar Dips
Regular Push-ups
Rest 60 seconds

STEP 2

Close Grip Pull-ups
Bar Dips
Diamond Push-ups
Rest 60 seconds

STEP 3

Reverse Grip Pull-ups
Bar Dips
Dive Bombers
Rest 60 seconds

STEP 4

Behind the Neck
Bar Dips
Regular Push-ups
Rest 60 seconds

STEP 5

Commandos
Bar Dips
Diamond Push-ups

I hope you enjoy and hate this routine as much as I do. You will see significant gains in your routine by applying this process to your workouts.

LEG BURN OUTS

STEP 1

The Wall
Frog Hops
Hand to Toe

STEP 2

Lunges
Star Hops
Side Sit-ups (Both sides)

STEP 3

Mountain Climbers
Atomics (Advanced)
Knee Bends (Beginner)

STEP 4

Fire Hydrant
High Knees
Crunches

STEP 5

Calf Raises
Sprints
Knee Roll Ups

You will see significant gains in your routine by applying this process to your workouts. SIGNIFICANT

Resolve to stop thinking negative thoughts such as "I can't—there's too much for me to overcome." Start saying *"I can! I will! Nobody will stop me!"* Each day is a new day and a new start, so make yours happen with SEAL Breakthrough Fitness.

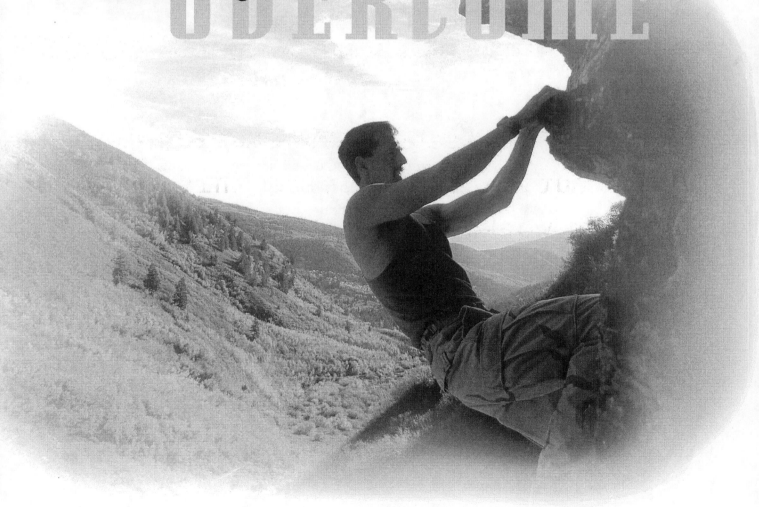

14

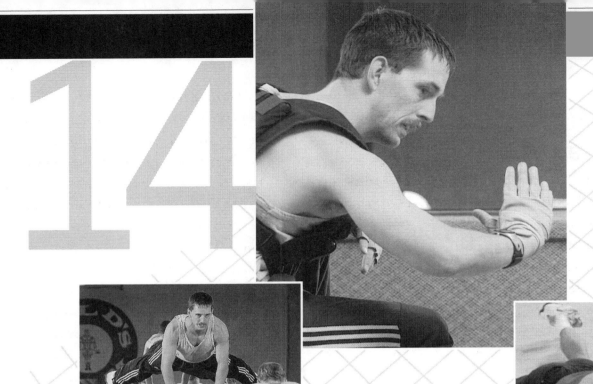

Concentrate on technique rather than repetitions.

CIRCUIT TRAINING AND TIMED INTERVALS

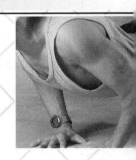

Into every routine you need to add diversity to your program. Anytime you can add changes that help you achieve your results without adding plateaus, go for it. Circuit training allows you to take everything you have learned, modify it, and push yourself to your limits. This shocks the body because you are taking it out of its comfort zone. Your body will shout, "What are you doing?" Don't listen too hard, for this will cause growth and changes.

Circuit training is a good time to concentrate on technique rather than repetitions. Everyone is guilty of trying to up their reps and qualify for the next level. It is our nature, whether we are male or female, to try to achieve more than we are physically capable of at the time. Even when we utilize the Pyramid or Blitzing Routines, we have a habit of wanting to get that extra rep in. This extra effort will cause you to break technique 90 percent of the time and block your progress.

In circuit training we are telling you, "OK, hard charger, just slow down and get back to basics. You will perform all the same exercises you have done previously but without repetitions. Repetitions will be exchanged for technique."

Perform each exercise with flawless technique and push yourself until you cannot go anymore. The minute you begin to compromise on technique, convert to the modified position or rest for 10 seconds and pick it up again. You are going to get tired, and you will not be able to go nonstop, so pay attention to your body. Focus inward and start to feel what your muscles are experiencing. Visualize every fiber in the muscle groups that you are working so that you can envision how they should be moving. Now slow your movement down and go for it!

CIRCUIT ROUTINES

BEGINNING ROUTINE

SET 1

Pull-ups (regular) — 5 reps
Bar Dips — 5 reps
Push-ups (regular) — 10 reps
Rest — 90 seconds

SET 2

Pull-ups (close grip) — 5 reps
Bar Dips — 5 reps
Push-ups (diamond) — 8 reps
Rest — 90 seconds

SET 3

Pull-ups (reverse grip) — 5 reps
Bar Dips — 5 reps
Push-ups (dive bombers) — 8 reps
Rest — 90 seconds

SET 4

Pull-ups (behind the neck) — 3 reps
Bar Dips — 5 reps
Push-ups (regular) — 8 reps
Rest — 90 seconds

INTERMEDIATE

SET 1

Pull-ups (regular) — 15 reps
Bar Dips — 20 reps
Push-ups (regular) — 40 reps
Rest — 30 seconds

SET 2

Pull-ups (close grip) — 15 reps
Bar Dips — 20 reps
Push-ups (diamond) — 30 reps
Rest — 30 seconds

SET 3

Pull-ups (reverse grip) — 15 reps
Bar Dips — 20 reps
Push-ups (dive bombers) — 30 reps
Rest — 30 seconds

SET 4

Pull-ups (behind the neck) — 10 reps
Bar Dips — 20 reps
Push-ups (regular) — 30 reps
Rest — 30 seconds

ADVANCED

SET 1

Pull-ups (regular) — 20 reps
Bar Dips — 30 reps
Push-ups (regular) — 60 reps
Rest — 30 seconds

SET 2

Pull-ups (close grip) — 20 reps
Bar Dips — 30 reps
Push-ups (diamond) — 40 reps
Rest — 30 seconds

SET 3

Pull-ups (reverse grip) — 20 reps
Bar Dips — 30 reps
Push-ups (dive bombers) — 40 reps
Rest — 30 seconds

SET 4

Pull-ups (behind the neck) — 15 reps
Bar Dips — 30 reps
Push-ups (regular) — 40 reps
Rest — 30 seconds

CIRCUIT TRAINING BY BODY PARTS

UPPER BODY	BEGINNING	INTERMEDIATE	ADVANCED
Exercise Duration	30 seconds	60 seconds	90 seconds

Regular Pull-ups
Close Grip Pull-ups
Reverse Grip Pull-ups
Commando Pull-ups
Behind the Neck Pull-ups
*Take a 30 second rest after each exercise.
**Take 60 second rest and drink some water.

BAR DIPS

One-minute's worth, then a 30 second rest.

PUSH-UPS

Regular Push-ups
Diamond Push-ups
Dive Bombers
*Take a 30 second rest after each exercise.
**Take 60 second rest and drink some water.

ABS — SHORT CONTRACTIONS

Short contractions through all the ab exercises. This means that there should be only a 2-inch difference between the contraction and return. For example, when you reach to touch your toes during Hand to Toes, as you come down you should only release two inches before you contract and then reach for your toes again.

Hand to Toes
Crunches
X Sit-ups
Side Sit-ups
Reverse Crunches
Hanging Leg Ups
Side Raises—Left side
Side Raises—Right side
*15 second rest in between all abdominal exercises.

LOWER BODY	BEGINNING	INTERMEDIATE	ADVANCED
Exercise Duration	30 seconds	60 seconds	90 seconds

Lunges
Squats
Calf Raises
   Regular
   Toe to Toe
   Heel to Heel
The Wall
Fire Hydrants

TIMED INTERVALS

Similar to Circuit Training, Timed Intervals are a tremendous way to work on technique because they allow you to focus on something other than repetitions. No matter how tired you get in this segment, focus completely on your form the entire time you are exercising. Use flawless form and go until you drop, then rest a few seconds and keep going until your time has finished.

You can use the exercises from the Circuit Training section. As long as you are systematically going from upper to lower body, you can switch around the exercises as to how you want within the muscle group. I recommend you do this section in front of a mirror so that you can watch your movements throughout the entire exercise.

During this section, be careful to time when you begin to fatigue and break technique. For example, perhaps you are performing at the beginning routine level, which is in 30 second intervals. At 45 seconds you begin to tire out and your form begins to give way to muscle failure. At the point your body begins to slow down, jot it down on a worksheet. Refer to this the next time you do the Timed Intervals and make it your goal to do one more perfect repetition after your last timed goal. Before you know it, you will find yourself performing way beyond your expectations in a shorter period of time.

I cannot emphasize enough that Circuit Training and Timed Intervals are a tremendous method to shake up your routine. These routines will keep your body in a constant state of shock, which in turn triggers proven growth and advancement. You can weave these routines in with your regular routine or every other month substitute it with your workout. Have fun and go do it!

" I cannot emphasize enough that Circuit Training and Timed Intervals are a tremendous method to shake up your routine. "

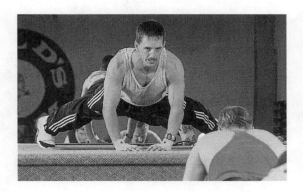

15

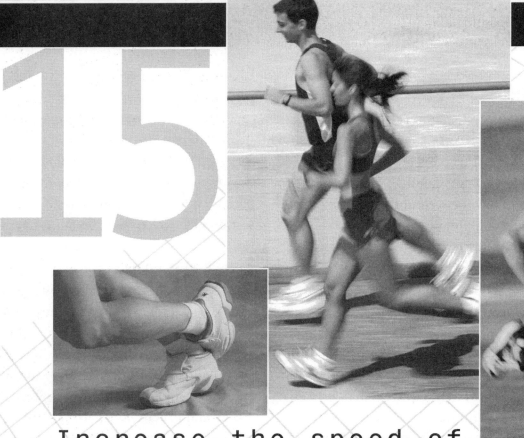

Increase the speed of
your strides—not the
length—to get faster.

RUNNING

Running is one of the most neglected and abused components in fitness routines. Far too many people in exercise programs focus exclusively on running long distance and end up overtraining and often hurting themselves. Our objective is to achieve a well-balanced workout, so keep everything in moderation while pushing yourself out of your comfort zones.

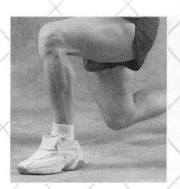

The key to your program is to find a perfect balance between working your short twitch muscles for quick burst running and your long twitch muscles for endurance running. You need to play around and become comfortable with both sprinting and long distance. Keep in mind that if you avoid running sprints or long distance because you dislike them, you're not going to achieve the optimum results you desire. Like anything else that requires growth and change, you need to push through what you dislike and get to your goal.

Marathon runners, you may not like this, but I have toned down the long-distance running program slightly and increased the sprinting. I have yet to meet a dedicated marathon runner who does not have knee or back injuries to go with their thousands of miles. We need endurance strength and stamina, but I think there's wisdom in shortening the distance while extending the frequency.

What we want is to find the perfect method for burning fat, maintaining our conditioning, while increasing our endurance in all areas. Remember to gradually work up to the levels you desire in each area of running. If you just go out there and start running mile after mile, day after day, something is going to give. I guarantee that you will burn yourself out and expose yourself to knee and back injuries. So listen to your body—it is the best indicator of what is or is not working.

Before you begin any running program, take a look at your gear. Running is very inexpensive, so don't try to save $20-30 on a cheap pair of running shoes that fail to give proper foot support and lead to a leg or foot injury. They must provide good heel support with an adequate sole

cushion. There should be a good balance in your shoes' flexibility, so avoid any sole that is too rigid or too flexible. Try to find a shoe store that specializes in athletic shoes and let them assist you in finding the right running shoes for your feet. Otherwise, go to our Web site at www.masterylevelfitness.com for recommended brands. You will be thankful in the end.

If you can't find a store with professionals who understand proper running shoes, I recommend having a partner run behind you to make sure you are not pronating too much. If your heels roll inward or outward too much, you are prone to knee and leg injuries. If the inside of your shoe is wearing away, it is a good indication that you are pronating. At the same time, you do not want to hit the surface of the ground too rigid. There are running shoes designed to help compensate for these problems. Find out what type of foot you have—high arch, low arch, wide or narrow foot. All these factors must be accounted for in the proper fitting of shoes and enjoyment of running. Also, get fitted for your shoes at the end of a day when your feet have swollen. Running shoes need to compensate for the fact that your feet will swell while you are running.

Another key to running is to find clothing that allows your skin to breathe. You want to feel as comfortable as possible when running or sprinting. Allow your pants/shorts to be elastic or flexible, and never wear a fabric that will rub your legs raw. During the winter months, wear fabrics that allow you to sweat, while at the same time extracting it from your body and keeping it off. Again, check out a good athletic store and familiarize yourself with these materials. Keeping your body dry and warm makes a huge difference in your running. Other gear that might make your cardio-routine more enjoyable and safe are heart rate monitors, portable radio/CD players, reflectors, and strap-on water bottles.

BEFORE YOU TAKE OFF

No matter how easy you intend your jog or run to be, always do at least 3-5 minutes of warm-up exercises prior to stretching. Then once you begin to stretch, spend at least five minutes of stretching the legs to bring them to master levels. Stretch all the muscle groups in your legs from the quadriceps to the calves and include your lower back in this routine. Do not forget to stretch after you finish your run or sprints. Flexibility is the name of the game.

I recommend waiting at least 90 minutes after a meal before you begin to exercise or run. To do so before then can cause stress on the heart, gastric discomfort, and impede the delivery of nutrients and oxygen to your vital organs.

POSITION

The key to running is to relax. It sounds elementary, but it's not always easy. Your foot should strike the ground first with the heel, roll to the ball of your feet, and explode off the toes. Try not to overstride, since this is hard on the knees, back, and hips. In sprinting I recommend having as soft a touch as possible in your stride. Think of how a gazelle seems to just glide over land. If you are hitting the ground hard during sprinting, you are not optimizing your form. You should barely hear the feet hit the ground. With long distance, slow your stride down and do not let your feet hit in front of your knees. In other words, your foot contact should occur in line

with the knee. Your leg should not be straight at the point of contact.

During long-distance runs, keep your back straight, head forward, and arms relaxed. During sprints your back should be at a slight tilt. Your arms should have a 90° bend. As you pump the left arm up (left arm should go out, then straight up), you should reach the height of your left ear. The right arm pumps back to the point that your right elbow is level with your right shoulder. If you are sprinting correctly, you will feel muscle fatigue in your triceps from this pumping motion. Next, lift with the quads, raise your knee to waist height, extend the feet out first then down. When it comes to long distance, the arms are completely relaxed with shorter rotations on the arm movements. Try not to clinch your fists while running long distance.

Increasing your long-distance running too fast can lead to injury. Do not increase your distance any more than 10-20 percent in any given week. And do not increase speed with distance. Do one or the other. Remember: You want to train smarter, not necessarily harder. In regards to frequency, there is no need to run more than 3-4 times a week. All exercise routines require time for your muscles to recover. When it comes to your intensity during long distance, use the "talk test." If you cannot hold a conversation with someone while running long distance, you have dropped into the anaerobic state. Sprints will take care of this for you, so you don't need to do so during aerobic exercise.

Hills present an incredible workout. If I want to get a quick burn and work the lungs, I hit the hills. If you truly want to increase your strength, speed, size, and endurance, incorporate hills into your training regimen. If you do not have hills nearby, go to your local high school or college for bleachers or find a local building that has several flights of stairs. Either way, definitely put sprinting uphill into your weekly routine. Take it easy coming down, though. No need to put added stress on the knees.

As you begin to sprint and run more often, increase your intake of antioxidants. The more you jog or run outside, the more pollutants you take in. So whether you get your antioxidants from natural foods or supplements, increase them. Also, increase your water intake. Drink at least a quart of water before leaving and a quart of water when you return. If your body weight drops more than 3 percent in any given day, you need to increase your water intake.

ENERGY CONSUMPTION

As you exercise, what affects your body's level of fatigue is how efficiently your body cells produce fuel. This is called the ATP process, which includes three systems that your body utilizes to produce fuel: anaerobic glycolysis, the creatine phosphate system, and the aerobic system.

The aerobic system is the dominant system of the body and requires oxygen. Whenever there are sufficient amounts of oxygen, the body will bypass the other two systems. However, when you begin to need quick burst energy or you get to a point where your body will not produce enough oxygen for its needs, the other two systems kick in.

The anaerobic glycolysis system requires no oxygen to break down the glycogen (glucose) stored in the muscles and liver, but this energy source is carried through the blood system and can only be maintained for a limited period of time. And though energy is released, lactic acid is also released as a byproduct, which inhibits the muscle performance. The more lactic acid produced, the less you are able to perform.

The creatine phosphate system provides quick burst energy. Creatine phosphate is a molecule that can be rapidly broken down to produce ATP. Unfortunately, even an Olympic athlete can only store enough creatine phosphate to last for 10 seconds.

Since there is a limited energy supply from these two secondary systems, your body's muscle groups can only maintain their intensity for a short period of time before fatigue sets in. The goal of our training is to push this point of fatigue (anaerobic threshold or lactate threshold) to its max so we can teach our body to use more and more of the aerobic system.

Another important factor is that the production in the ATP process involves several complex chemicals. Carbohydrates and fats are two of the primary elements used in this process. When your body is at rest, it mostly uses fatty acids and glucose in the ATP process. It is the level of your physical conditioning that determines the percentage of fatty acids-to-glucose used. The better your physical condition, the more your body taps into fatty acids. As your exercise routine intensifies, your body expands its ability to produce more ATP through the aerobic system. Nevertheless, you will eventually get to a point where your body will not produce enough oxygen for its needs and will switch to the anaerobic.

Besides lactic acid, hyperventilation is another form that the body uses to indicate lack of ATP production. In actuality, hyperventilation is not a cure for lack of oxygen. VO_2 max is what determines the capacity of your body's ability to consume oxygen. VO_2 has two major factors—the ability to deliver and to extract oxygen from the blood.

VO_2 max = maximum cardio output X maximum oxygen extracted

VO_2 = volume of oxygen consumed

Through training we are going to increase the anaerobic threshold point, and we will push your VO_2 max to increase your aerobic capabilities.

A generic rule of thumb for burning fat is to keep your cardio sessions to a minimum of 30-45 minutes in order to tap into your fat cells. Otherwise, you may be helping your muscles but not optimizing your body's metabolism clock.

RUNNING ROUTINES

As we cover sprinting, long distance, and interval training, I provide guidelines, but you will have the flexibility to design your own routines. Let's start out with sprinting.

SPRINTING

Start out with cone training. Set up your cones in 20-yard increments. These cones will be used in acceleration sprints as well as interval training. This program works best at a school track of 400 yards.

BEGINNING LEVEL

Warm up by running 800 yards at a nice even pace. Set 3 cones at intervals of 20 yards apart.

Accelerations: Run the first 20 yards at 50 percent speed (easy pace) and begin getting into full sprint position. Take the second 20 yards at 75 percent speed, and the third 20 yards at 100 percent speed.

Do a total of 5 sets of cones.

INTERMEDIATE LEVEL

Do everything the same as the beginning level but increase your sets to 10.

ADVANCED

Do everything the same as the beginning level but increase your sets to 20.

- It is important to keep a running log of your progress while using acceleration exercises.
- If you have a friend who can help you out, have them log your times between each cone. As you learn to increase your times, your overall speed will naturally become faster.
- There are stopwatches that allow you to stop times during each cone, yet give you an overall time for the full 60 yards.
- Accelerations are where I really want you to concentrate on your running technique. Technique can make or break your times in this program.

INTERVAL SPRINTS

Four cones will be needed for this exercise. At the straightaway on each end of the track, I want you to place cones. You will begin this exercise at the beginning of the track where it curves. Start out jogging, then when you reach the straightaway begin your sprints. Do not end your sprints until you reach the end of the straightaway.

BEGINNING LEVEL

Run 2 laps of 400 yards = 800 yards

INTERMEDIATE LEVEL

Run 6 laps of 400 yards = 2,400 yards (1.5 miles)

ADVANCED LEVEL

Run 8 laps of 400 yards = 3,200 yards (2 miles)

This same process can be done in your neighborhood. Just measure the distance with your vehicle or sprint down one end of the street and jog back the other. Keep track of the times no matter whether it is the street or track. This will be your indictor as to when you are ready to advance to the next level or not.

LONG DISTANCE

As mentioned before, I have toned down the distances in this book. I want you to still push yourself when it comes to distances and times, but give yourself sufficient time to rest.

BEGINNING LEVEL

Monday	1 mile
Wednesday	1 mile
Friday	1 mile
Alternative	
Tuesday	1 mile
Thursday	1 mile
Saturday	1 mile (*optional*)

INTERMEDIATE LEVEL

Monday	3 miles
Wednesday	3 miles
Friday	3 miles
Alternative	
Tuesday	3 miles
Thursday	3 miles
Saturday	3 miles (*optional*)

ADVANCED LEVEL

Monday	6 miles
Wednesday	6 miles
Friday	6 miles
Alternative	
Tuesday	6 miles
Thursday	6 miles
Saturday	6 miles

COMBINED

Monday	6 miles
Wednesday	2 miles accelerations or interval sprints
Friday	6 miles

Tuesday/Thursday/Saturday— same as **Monday/Wednesday/Friday**

I recommend that you switch your sprints around every other week to reach Master Level conditioning.

Week 1—Accelerations.

Week 2—Intervals.

16

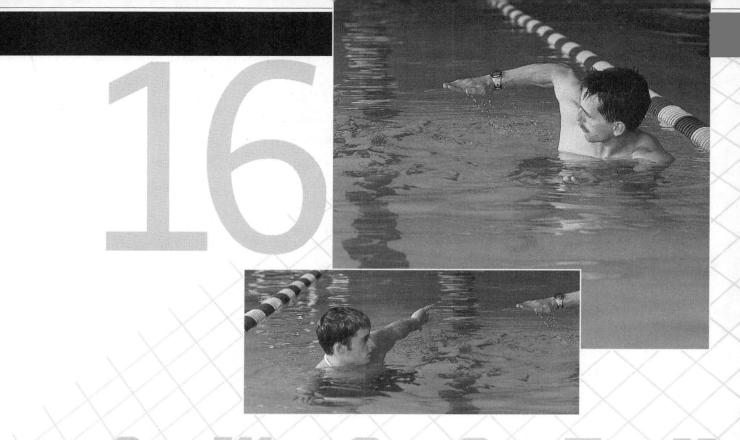

Remember, *smooth is fast.*

S M O O T H

SWIMMING

I f you truly want to see great results in your cardio-routine along with resistance, then try incorporating swimming in your routine. Swimming provides an incredible workout without taking a heavy toll on the body. The buoyancy that you get in the water takes a lot of pressure off your joints. As you glide through the water and push the water with arm strokes and leg kicks, you instantly feel the resistance throughout your entire body.

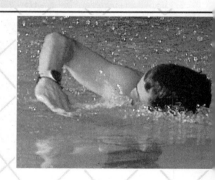

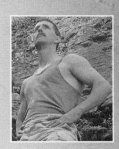

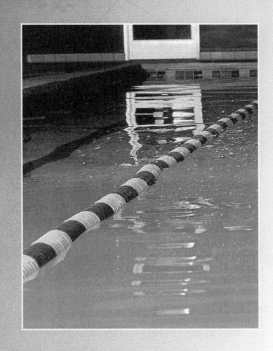

"Add up the benefits. You receive cardio results, resistance results, increased stamina and strength, yet you avoid putting pressure on your joints."

Add up the benefits. You receive cardio results, resistance results, increased stamina and strength, yet you avoid putting pressure on your joints. It does require extra effort to take advantage of swimming, but it's worth scheduling it into even a busy lifestyle. If you have the luxury of working out near a pool, take advantage of it.

To become successful in the water and maximize the workout benefits, you have to learn to master your lungs and breathing. Otherwise, you will never feel comfortable enough to enjoy the workout. Swimming is a cardio workout, and you are going to feel it in every major muscle group as well as simultaneously feel it in your lungs. You must learn to control and mentally slow your breathing down, which will allow you to increase your distance while maintaining a sense of comfortableness. Whether I am running or swimming, I keep telling myself to slow my breathing frequency. With training you can actually learn to master yourself and manually control your respiration. It's simply a matter of learning to improve your technique.

STROKE

Your stroke is the key to success in the pool. It begins with the proper hand formation. Pretend as though you are reaching for a sip of water out of your hands. The formation you make with your cupped hands is exactly the form you need in the water. Now, separate your hands but maintain the cup formation with each hand. Next, your arm strokes must be fluid and smooth. There is no reason to slap the water or thrust them recklessly. As you reach out in front of yourself with your right hand, extend your arm as far as you possibly can. Once you have reached your full extension, the palm of your

hand should be facing down into the water. With a strong thrust, push your hand forcefully downward into the water. On the upward movement your hand should brush the outside of your hip. Your palm should be facing up, getting ready to exit the water.

As your hand exits the water, reverse the position of your palm so that it is facing the water again. The forward movement of your hand should be treated like an arrow skimming over the top of the water. Do not drag your full arm completely out of the water and then shove it back in again. Your hand should only rise out of the water about 3-4 inches, then smoothly glide across the surface and enter softly at the end of your extension. There should not be any splash when it reenters the water, and there really should not be much splash when it exits.

Remember: *Smooth is fast*. Many people think that the faster they move their arms or legs through the water, the faster they will swim. But someone with a good, smooth technique can swim at half the arm and leg velocity and still blow past that person. Break the old thoughts that your arms and legs propel you through the water. Swimming is a full-body movement, and until you understand that, you will never become proficient in the water.

Think of your body as a torpedo in the water and keep your movements as close to the body as possible. Every move needs to be as streamlined as possible, which is why your arm stroke goes straight down while brushing your hips as it comes up. To help your body stay more streamline, lean slightly on your chest to maintain your legs and hips near the surface. If you let your legs drop too deep in the water, you begin to drag rather than slice through the water. To maintain proper form you must achieve a balance between legs and arms. I cannot emphasize enough to concentrate on technique not speed, because if you improve technique, speed will naturally follow.

SWIMMING ROUTINES

BEGINNING LEVEL

This routine will give you the basic routines to help you achieve Master Level cardio fitness. Simply alternate Part I and Part II every other week.

Part I = week 1
Part II = week 2
Part I = week 3
Part II = week 4

PART I

Monday—Stroke (Freestyle) — 500 yards

Wednesday—Stroke (Freestyle) — 500 yards

Friday—Stroke (Sidestroke) — 750 yards

PART II

Monday—Stroke (Freestyle) Intervals — 50 yards sprint/100 yards relaxed Pace = 500 yards

Wednesday—Stroke (Sidestroke) — 750 yards

Friday—Stroke (Freestyle) Intervals — 50 yards sprint/100 yards relaxed Pace = 500 yards

INTERMEDIATE LEVEL

PART I

Monday—Stroke (Freestyle) — 1,500 yards

Wednesday—Stroke (Freestyle) — 1,500 yards

Friday—Stroke (Sidestroke) — 2,000 yards

PART II

Monday—Stroke (Freestyle) Intervals — 100 yards sprint/200 yards relaxed Pace = 1,500 yards

Wednesday—Stroke (Sidestroke) — 2,000 yards

Friday—Stroke (Freestyle) Intervals — 100 yards Sprint/200 yards relaxed Pace = 1,500 yards

ADVANCED LEVEL

PART I

Monday—Stroke (Freestyle) — 5,200 yards

Wednesday—Stroke (Freestyle) — 5,200 yards

Friday—Stroke (Sidestroke) — 6,400 yards

PART II

Monday—Stroke (Freestyle) Intervals — 200 yards/400 yards relaxed pace = 3,200 yards

Wednesday—Stroke (Sidestroke) — 6,400 yards

Friday—Strokes (Freestyle) Intervals — 200 yards/400 yards relaxed Pace = 3,200 yards

•This routine can also be switched to Tuesday, Thursday, and Saturday.

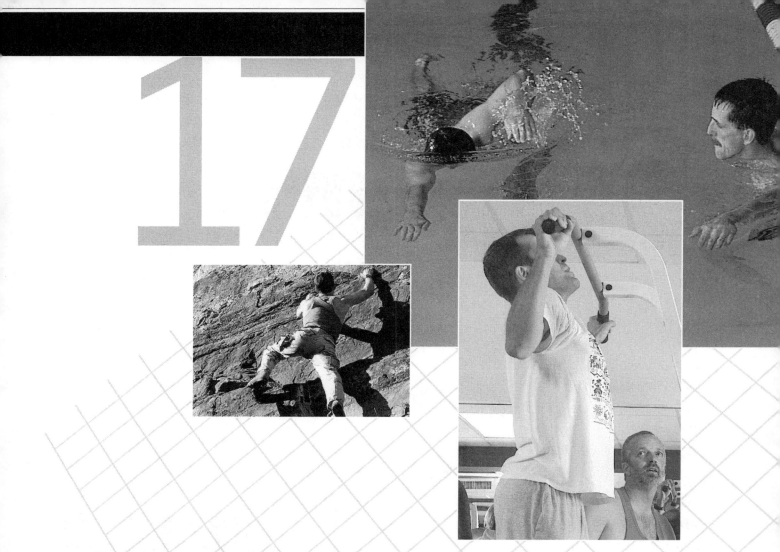

17

Versatility

COMBINING

Nothing can compensate for versatility. In the combined routines we are simply applying routines from the running and swimming sections to add one complete routine. This would be the ultimate routine to follow for Master Level Fitness. Once again, this is the routine you would substitute for your cardio days.

Monday

SUNDAY	MONDAY	TUESDAY	WEDNESDAY	THURSDAY	FRIDAY	SATURDAY

Friday

Wednesday

BEGINNING LEVEL

Week 1

Monday—Accelerations — 800 yards

Wednesday—Freestyle — 1,000 yards

Friday—Long Distance — 1 mile

Week 2

Monday—Accelerations — Hill Sprints for 5 minutes

Wednesday—Side Stroke — 1,000 yards

Friday—Long Distance — 1 mile

INTERMEDIATE LEVEL

Week 1

Monday—Accelerations — 2,400 yards

Wednesday—Freestyle — 1,600 yards

Friday—Long Distance — 3 miles

Week 2

Monday—Accelerations — Hill Sprints for 10 minutes

Wednesday—Side Stroke — 1,600 yards

Friday—Long Distance — 3 miles

ADVANCED LEVEL

Week 1

Monday—Accelerations — 3,200 yards

Wednesday—Freestyle — 3,200 yards

Friday—Long Distance — 6 miles

Week 2

Monday—Accelerations — Hill Sprints for 15 minutes•

Wednesday—Side Stroke — 3,200 yards

Friday—Long Distance — 6 miles

Hill Sprints can be substituted with bleachers, stairs, etc.

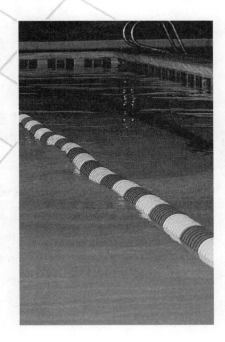

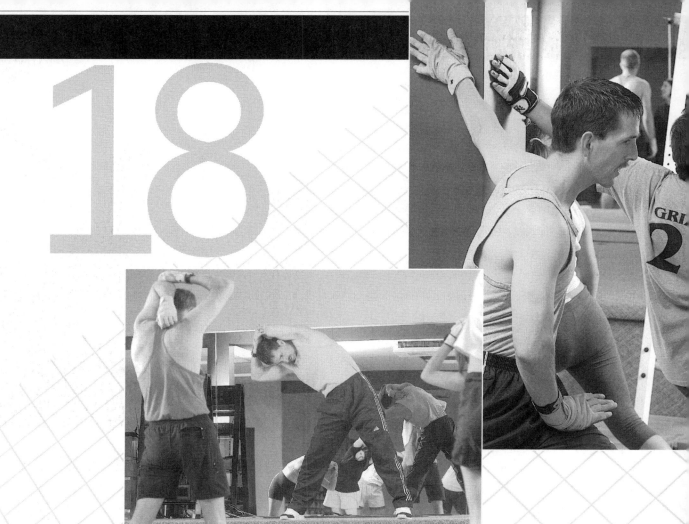

stret

COOL DOWN WITH STRETCHING

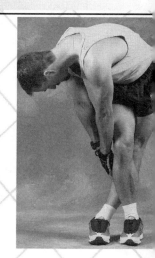

Do not take your cool downs for granted. Far too often we close our exercise routine with a swish of the forehead and a pat on the back, then we pick up our gear and go home. You do deserve a pat on the back, but you're not finished. One of the most important aspects of our routine is next. You must take the short amount of time it takes to stretch and properly let your body cool down. Immediately after you finish your routine, go ahead and walk around for approximately 2 minutes to bring your heart rate back down. I don't know about you, but when I push myself hard and start to feel nauseous, the last thing I want to do is bend over and place my hands on my thighs. That only makes the upset stomach worse. I highly recommend you keep your hands on your hips, your head and chin high. Stick out that old chest of yours and let some fresh air come into your lungs.

Next, after your heart rate has come down and you feel a little more relaxed, sit down and begin to stretch for about 5-10 minutes. Remember that the best time for increasing flexibility is to stretch after your exercise routine. It will also help reduce the soreness you might normally feel the next day. I also highly recommend stretching on your off days, which helps in the muscle tightness.

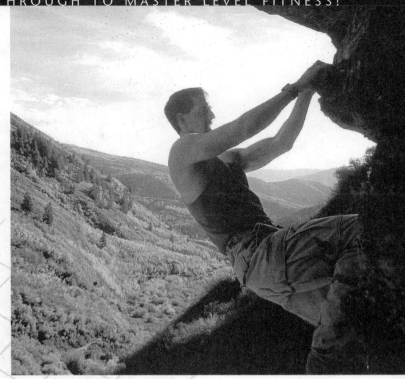

Increase flexibility!

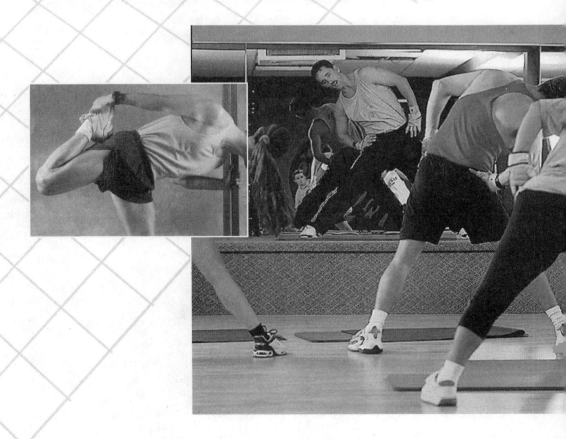

19

NUTRITION

BY BROOKE ISAAKSON

In the United States, where 16 million adults struggle with diabetes and over half the adult population is considered overweight, proper nutrition and exercise may save your life. The Senate Select Committee on Human Needs established the Dietary Goals for the United States in 1977. This was the first recommendation for health promotion rather than just focusing on deficiency. Those guidelines were reviewed and changed in 1995 to the Dietary Guidelines for Americans, which are general suggestions for all healthy Americans who are over the age of two.

THE DIETARY GUIDELINES FOR AMERICANS

The *Dietary Guidelines for Americans* pamphlet recommends that people "diet with most of the calories from grain products, vegetables, fruits, low fat milk products, lean meats, fish, poultry, and dry beans." The four food groups they suggest are legumes, fruits, vegetables, and milk. If you focus on these categories, your diet will naturally have a lot less fat and calories. Meat should be eaten sparingly, versus every day for every meal. By focusing on legumes (kidney, garbanzo, refried, and black beans, etc.) and other sources of protein, such as nuts and seeds, you will be much healthier.

The ABCs of a healthy lifestyle are outlined as:
Aim for Fitness
- Aim for a healthy weight.
- Be physically active each day.

Build a Healthy Base
- Let the Food Guide Pyramid direct your food choices.
- Choose a variety of grains daily, especially whole grains.
- Choose a variety of fruits and vegetables daily.
- Keep food safe to eat.

Choose sensibly
- Choose a diet that is low in saturated fat and cholesterol and moderate in total fat.
- Choose beverages and foods to moderate your intake of sugars.
- Choose and prepare food with less salt.

Do you know how to translate nutrition lingo such as RDAs (Recommended Daily Allowances), Dietary Guidelines, and Daily Values into practical use? RDAs refer to nutrients needed to meet the needs of most healthy people. The Dietary Guidelines describe food choices that will help meet these recommendations mentioned in detail (the ABCs). The Daily Values are based on a 2,000-calorie diet. The Nutrition Facts labels (on most foods) and the Food Guide Pyramid are tools that put the Dietary Guidelines into practice. The Pyramid makes the RDAs and the Dietary Guidelines into types and amounts of food to consume each day. Although these tools are easily available, few Americans utilize them. About 55 percent of Americans are considered obese, and some are consuming 60 percent of their diet from fats and oils.

ENERGY SOURCES AND FATS

So how do we translate this information into real life? First, we must understand where our main energy sources come from. Primarily, we need 55-60 percent of our energy from carbohydrates. Carbohydrates are the quick energy source and come from starches such as potatoes, simple sugars such as honey and table sugar, and complex carbohydrates such as whole grain breads, fruits, and vegetables. If the body is not getting enough carbohydrates, it will go into a state of ketosis, which means that ketone bodies are accumulating in the blood. High ketone levels can result in coma and death. The body has to have glucose (from carbs) for energy first and foremost.

Second, protein needs are about 10-20 percent. This can vary with individual activity and needs. Protein is important for repair and many other body functions, but it should not come close to carbohydrate consumption. Protein use in excess will be excreted in the urine or turned into fat. Protein has 4 kcal per gram.

Fat is the final source of energy requiring less than 25 percent of our energy needs. Many nutritionists recommend 15-25 percent of energy from fat. Fat is essential for many bodily functions. It rounds out body contours, protects vital organs, provides stored energy (9 kcal/gram), and insulates the body from changes in temperature.

Most Americans receive their fat intake from animal sources, which are saturated fats. One main characteristic of saturated fats is that they are solid at room temperature. Diets high in saturated fats increase LDL cholesterol, which results in heart disease. Meat is a wonderful source of iron, zinc, creatine, protein, etc., but also very fatty. The American Heart Association and the National Cattleman's Beef Association suggest choosing lean meats and trimming the fat before cooking. Calories, fat, and cholesterol can be greatly reduced by trimming all external fat and removing the skin from poultry.

Stay away from trans-fatty acids, which are a form of monounsaturated fat. These are the worst types of fat and are used to stabilize a product for longer store shelf life. Hydrogenation is the term used to describe the process of stabilization, so watch out and limit these fats. Trans-fatty acids are in fast foods, peanut butter, and vegetable shortening, among others. One alternative would be natural peanut butter.

Americans tend to forget to focus on monounsaturated and polyunsaturated fats. Based on a 2,000-calorie diet, only 65g of total fat should be consumed with 20g or less from saturated fats. Based on the 25 percent rule of energy from fat, 8.33 percent should be saturated, 8.33 percent monounsaturated, and 8.33 percent polyunsaturated. If percentages are lower, adjust your figures.

What food sources provide the "good" fats? Monounsaturated fatty acids are commonly found in the form of olive and canola oils (oleic acid) and may be protective against cardiovascular disease. Monounsaturated fat is liquid at room temperature and cloudy in your refrigerator. There are two types of dietary polyunsaturated fats: Omega-6 and Omega-3. These are called the essential fatty acids because they cannot be produced in the body. Omega-6 helps reduce LDL cholesterol, but high consumption also decreases HDL, the "good" cholesterol that helps reduce the risk of heart disease. Omega-3 helps reduce LDL, but also increases HDL. Omega-6 (alphalinolenic acid) is found in vegetable oils and fish oils. It is better to get your Omega-3 from sources such as salmon and albacore tuna as opposed to supplements. Most Americans don't have an Omega-6 deficiency problem, yet Omega-3 is much harder for them to acquire in their diet.

DIET AND EXERCISE

To diet or not to diet, that is the question. I believe that diets do not work because they are too restrictive and cannot be applied for the rest of your life. There are no "bad" foods, but you need to consume foods that meet your nutrient needs while supplying energy and satiety. You can eat what you want, but you must do it in moderation. One food choice is not going to make or break your diet. Just balance out your choices throughout the day or even during the week so that overall consumption is adequate and healthy. Apply diversity to your diet, or boredom will set in, which sets you up for bingeing. Foods that differ in color, texture, temperature, and taste keep things interesting.

Did you know that there are 3,500 kilocalories in one pound of fat? So to lose one pound, 3,500 calories must be lost. Only one-half to one pound of weight loss per week is suggested for healthy and prolonged weight loss. Up to two pounds per week is the suggested limit. To break down the calories per week, 500 calories must be burned off per day. The best way to lose weight is to exercise consistently, applying cardio, resistance training, and stretching to your workout. Limiting the number of calories consumed is not suggested, just the types of foods consumed. For example, if you now eat a box of Krispy Kreme donuts for breakfast, a Big Mac and fries for lunch, and a 12-ounce steak and potatoes for dinner, there are many possibilities for change. Vegetables and fruits need to be added along with low-fat milk products, whole grain breads, and a lot of water.

Decrease the amount of high fat, low nutrient foods for better health. Remember to follow the Food Guide Pyramid indefinitely. No one food group is less or more important than another. The USDA's Center for Nutrition Policy and Promotion list three basic steps for losing weight: (1) Increase physical activity, (2) Reduce fat and sugars in your diet, and (3) Stick with the Food Guide Pyramid, reducing intake to the lowest amount of servings suggested.

Not everyone needs the same amount of calories, especially at different stages of life. There are three basic categories of calorie intake to set some guidelines. If you are a sedentary woman, or for some older adults, 1,600 calories a day is proposed. For most children (over age two), teenage girls, active women, and many sedentary men, 2,200 calories are suggested. If you are a teenage boy, active man, or very active woman, 2,800 calories is about right. Pregnant and lactating women need at least 2,200 calories, but may need more.

Below are sample diets for a day at the three calorie levels from the USDA's Center for Nutrition Policy and Promotion. The numbers represent amount of servings unless otherwise indicated.

	LOWER ABOUT 1,600	MIDDLE ABOUT 2,200	HIGH ABOUT 2,800
GRAIN GROUP	6	9	11
VEGETABLE GROUP	3	4	5
FRUIT GROUP	2	3	4
MILK GROUP	2-3*	2-3*	2-3*
MEAT GROUP	5	6	7
TOTAL FAT	53 GRAMS	73 GRAMS	93 GRAMS
TOTAL ADDED SUGARS	6 TSP.	12 TSP.	18 TSP.

*Teenagers, young adults to age 24, and pregnant and lactating women need 3 servings.

THE ESSENTIAL ROLE OF WATER

Water is essential for survival, but why? Water does not provide energy, but it is irreplaceable because the body cannot store water. Water regulates many functions in the body. Blood is 90 percent water, and it transports nutrients and oxygen to cells, lubricates and cleans, and protects during pregnancy. Water is a regulator of temperature, is involved in chemical reactions, and is a solvent. Water intake must equal water loss in order to maintain homeostasis.

The body sends out many clues when it needs water. A person's saliva decreases, making your throat dry and initiating the need for water consumption. The increased need for water causes a decrease in overall blood volume and a lowered blood pressure. The brain senses this need, but this is not a fail-proof regulator. If you are thirsty, the actual need for water is lagging. While exercising, drink 3-6 ounces of water every 15 minutes to ensure balance of water in the body. The basic daily suggestion for water intake is 8-10 cups (8 ounces) daily. Physical activity, especially in the heat, and dieting require much more. As crude as it may sound, the SEAL Teams were taught to watch the color of their urine. Coming from the desert team, they were constantly training in hot environments, and by keeping their urine clear and not yellow, they were able to ensure proper hydration.

When dieting, drinking a lot of water helps eliminate fat. Dr. Donald S. Robertson wrote an article entitled "How 8 Glasses a Day Keep Fat Away" that has gotten all over Internet health and fitness Web sites. He points out that water suppresses the appetite and helps the body metabolize stored fat. Studies have indicated that an increase in water intake can actually reduce fat deposits. If you have problems with retaining fluid, increased water intake actually lessens the retention. When the body receives less water than needed, it perceives this as a need to store, which shows up as swollen legs, hands, and feet. Water aids the body in the elimination of waste. This action is particularly useful when dieting, because of the need for elimination of excess waste. Dr. Robertson suggests while dieting to increase water intake to 12 cups a day. The schedule he proposes is as follows:

Morning: 1 quart (4 cups) over a minute period.

Noon: 1 quart consumed over a minute period.

Evening: 1 quart consumed between 5 & 6 P.M.

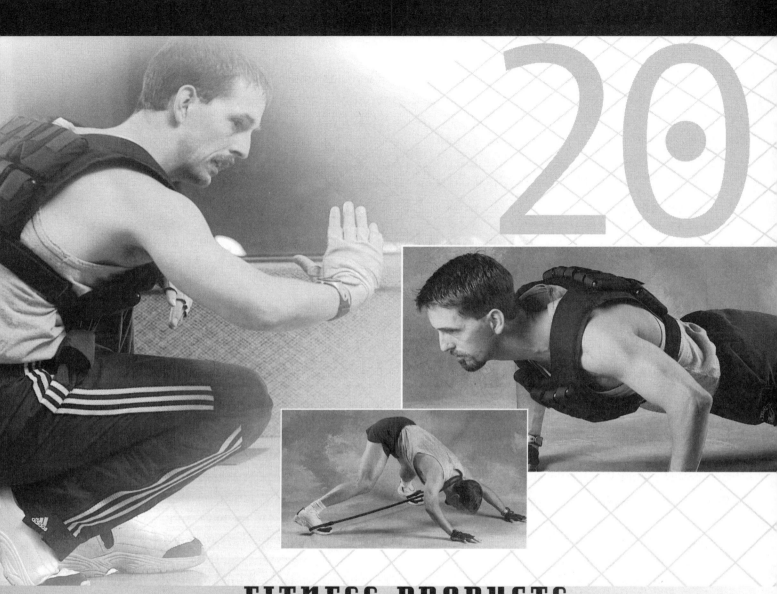

FITNESS PRODUCTS

Any routine can become tired or boring, even a great workout. Perhaps your body has reached a plateau and you need something new to jump-start it. I have found a few items that are of high quality and bring tremendous versatility to a workout. Whether you want to gain more muscle mass or just shock the body to keep it in a state of growth, I recommend you consider the following products.

POWER PUSH-UP

I have not found a more durable or better-built product that utilizes resistance bands than the *Power Push-up*. It allows you to generate more resistance while performing basic or complicated push-ups. You do not have to worry about outgrowing this product either. With the ability to interchange bands or add one at a time, your resistance can always be modified. One important tip: Keep the band that goes around your back as high as possible. You do not want the band to slide down into the lower back region and add stress to this area.

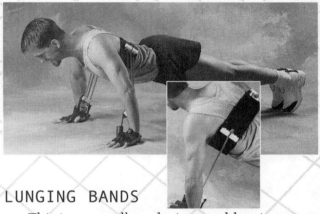

LUNGING BANDS

This is an excellent device to add resistance to your lunges and Dive Bomber push-ups. Simply slip your feet into each handgrip while placing

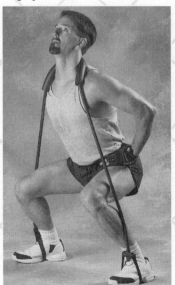

the foam pad around your neck. Instantly you will feel the resistance as you extend down underneath the fence. At the same time you will feel the bands wanting to bring you back to your original position, which is where you have to fight the urge to cheat. To get full benefit out of your *Power Bands,* you must slow your movement from the full extension position back to the starting position.

For lunges, keep the band in the same position. Your body will not be as stable as you were without the bands. Keep your movements slow and methodical to avoid falling off balance. Any time you slow down your movements, the focus changes from reps to technique.

WEIGHT VEST

The weight vest will allow you to perform a wide range of exercises without having to change devices or positions of the device. This weight vest can be modified in increments of 2 pounds and goes up to 50 pounds. By simply adjusting the Velcro belt, the vest fits nice and snug. Do not wear the vest too loose, as the vest may slide around on your body. Your body can also receive a pounding effect as you perform fast movement exercises. This is a very durable product, and the weights are difficult to damage.

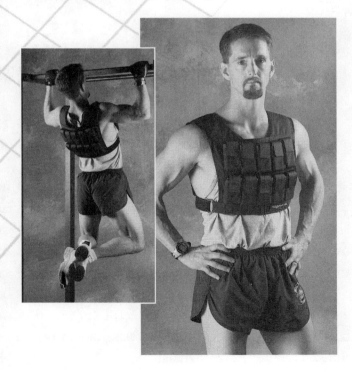

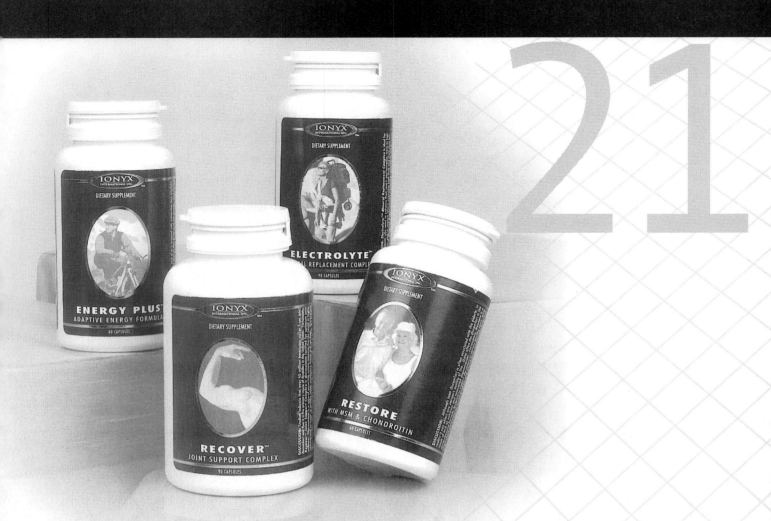

21

IONYX CUTTING-EDGE MINERAL SUPPLEMENTATION

Proper supplementation of key nutrients is critical for one's body to function at peak performance while exercising. When you perspire, you lose more than water to cool your overheated body. You also lose important electrolytes (essential minerals) that help control fluid levels in the body, maintain normal pH levels, and ensure the correct electric potential between nerve cells, which enables the proper transmission of nerve signals.

Minerals are a key to a person's overall good health because 95 percent of the body's daily functions require them. Our bodies cannot produce minerals, so they must be ingested through the foods and liquids we consume. Unfortunately, eating the right foods is no longer good enough because the mineral content of our foods is on the decline. If you compare the 1963 and 1997 United States Department of Agriculture Nutrition Tables, most of the trace and essential minerals in our fruits, vegetables, and meats have decreased considerably. The loss varies from 20 to 85 percent on any given mineral, and wisdom tells you that supplementation is necessary to avoid deficiency, especially if you work out.

I never realized how important minerals were until I started using a phenomenal electrolyte product from IONYX International, Inc., which uses a unique formula that replaces the electrolytes lost during intense workouts. I take their electrolyte supplement every day before I exercise, and I've had amazing results. I found that I have more energy during the workout and am able to perform longer without the muscle fatigue that normally kicks in. That enables me to press the fatigue threshold and perform at a higher level. I also discovered that my muscle recovery was much quicker, since I was replenishing the minerals my body sweats out.

When I compared the IONYX products to others on the market, they have no equal. The minerals from IONYX are the most bio-available because they are the smallest in size. They have natural assimilative properties, so they do not need to be put into a solution or have other ingredients attached to them to be absorbed into your body. They have pH balancing characteristics that are more concentrated than other supplements.

I am not the only one who has seen amazing results using the IONYX supplements. George Curtis, the head athletic trainer for the athletic programs at Brigham Young University, put his athletes on the IONYX supplements. After they became the only university that had all five fall sports programs ranked in the national top 20, here's what Curtis had to say:

"We have had an ongoing problem for years trying to find the right combination of electrolytes to take with our combination of drinks. It has been a real difficult task. We have tried all kinds of combinations, but this spring when we tried IONYX products it was great to see how much they eased the problem with some of the chronic problems athletes had. We will be exclusively buying the IONYX Electrolyte supplements over other previous products."

Another individual who has had great results using IONYX supplements with his athletes is David Houle, head coach for Mountain View High School and national high school Coach of the Year 2000, who has won 57 state championships throughout his career coaching basketball and track and field. When he gave the IONYX products to his kids, listen to these results:

"For the past couple of months I have been sampling a product by the name of IONYX. I have had athletes from various sports that I coach try this product, and they have found it to be very beneficial. It is a natural product that helps kids with their stamina. I have witnessed some of my athletes break personal, state, and national records using IONYX products. Clearly, I am excited about this product line and what it can do to help the quality of our everyday lives."

If you do not replenish your electrolytes while exercising, your body may suffer fatigue, low stamina, muscle cramping, lack of recovery, and even invite disaster! The electrolyte supplement from IONYX is ideal for anyone who experiences high fluid and electrolyte loss, and I recommend it completely.

For more information about these electrolyte supplements or to find out how to purchase IONYX products, please refer to my Web site at www.masterlevelfitness.com.

PRE-WORKOUT SUPPLEMENTS

ELECTROLYTE™ Mineral Replacement Complex: When individuals perspire, they lose more than water to cool their overheated body. They also lose precious electrolytes (essential minerals). Our unique formula replaces not only the common electrolytes needed for peak performance, but the ionic minerals that are commonly overlooked when electrolyte replacement is considered. If individuals do not replenish their electrolytes, their body may suffer fatigue, low stamina, muscle cramping, lack of recovery, and even invite disaster! This complex is ideal for those individuals who need to enhance their sports performance, or when they experience high fluid and electrolyte loss. (Take 3 capsules before each workout.)

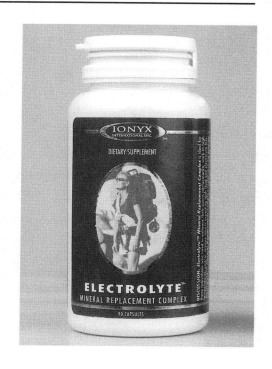

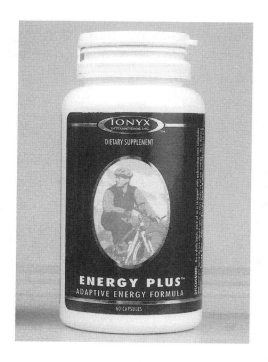

ENERGY PLUS™ Adaptive Energy Formula: This complex increases one's energy level during stressful and intense workouts. Siberian and Korean Ginseng help one's body to withstand adverse physical and mental conditions during cases of weakness, exhaustion, and tiredness, while improving mental alertness. Guarana provides extra stamina and endurance, increases strength, reduces fatigue, and helps dispose the body of lactic acid, which builds up in the muscles and causes muscle fatigue. Vitamin B complex is essential for maintaining energy levels and ensuring long-lasting performance. (Take 3 capsules before each workout.)

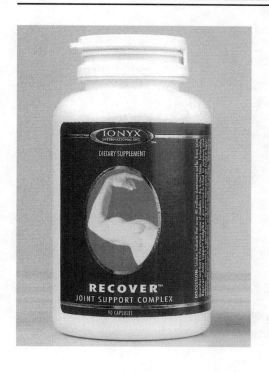

RECOVER™ Joint Support Complex: When one is constantly building and developing stamina and endurance, it is critical to not overlook the importance of fortifying one's body with the nutrients needed for optimum joint wellness. Common "wear and tear" can be minimized with proper supplementation. Glucosamine, in combination with other supportive ingredients in this formula, nourish one's body so it can repair itself and return its joints to proper health. While many drugs are used to fight against joint discomfort, they regrettably only target the symptoms and do very little to address the actual problem. Glucosamine, on the other hand, is a natural aminomonosaccaride found in high concentrated amounts in healthy joints, connective tissues, and cartilage. As a result, this formula is the better long-term choice for healthy joints. (Take 3 capsules before each workout.)

RESTORE™ With MSM & Chondroitin: This unique formula is a synergistic blend of MSM, Chondroitin, and other beneficial herbs, which provide the building blocks for the body to repair its joints. MSM assists the body in healing and repairing many of its tissues, especially those at risk of repeated damage. Chondroitin is a major constituent found in cartilage that helps form holes within the matrix of one's joints, which the body fills with water, creating a spongy shock absorber for the joints. (Take 2 capsules before each workout.)

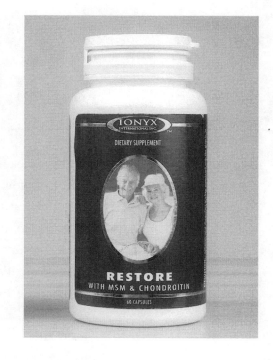

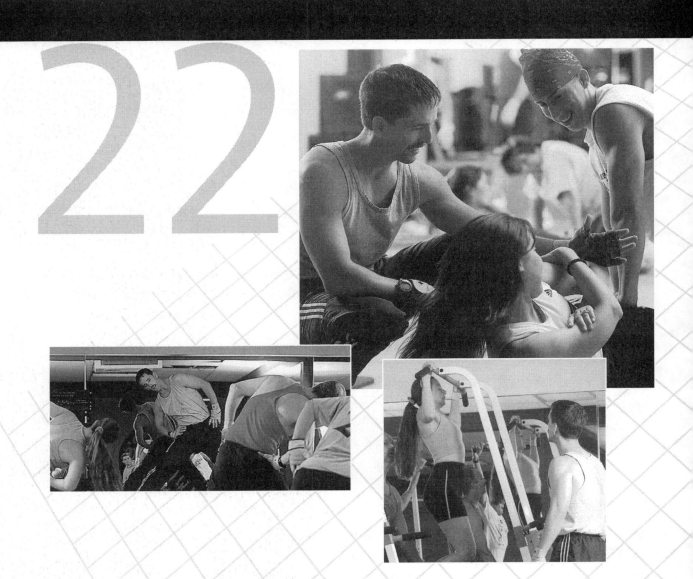

22

CONCLUSION

The Master Level program is laid out in an easy-to-follow and easy-to-use format. We have even created a 12-week workbook, so there is no excuse as to what to do. Each day you just check off what is required, and in three months you will see a transformation. You're going to have fun because the program works, and you'll be pleased with the results. Take it one day at a time and do not bite off more than you can chew. Be realistic and refuse to set yourself up for failure by setting lofty goals. And when you do accomplish your goals, pat yourself

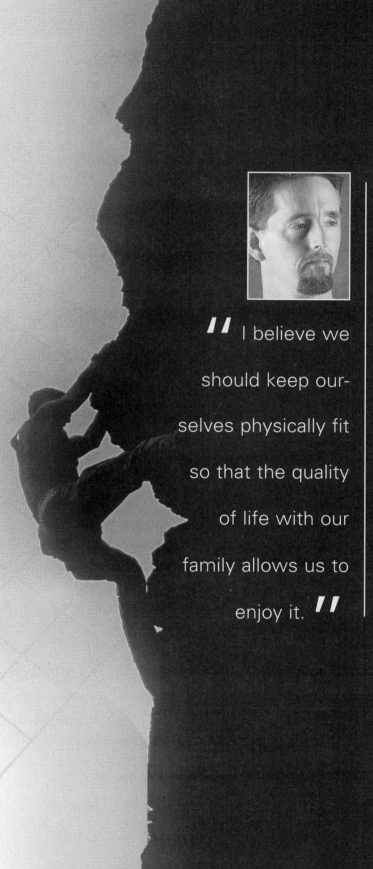

on the back. This does not mean you head off to get a burger when you lose the first two pounds.

With the Master Level program, you are going to experience phenomenal changes in muscle density, endurance, strength, and power. It encompasses everything from fast-twitch muscles to slow-twitch. But you will only get out of it what you put into it. In other words, if you only perform 50 percent of the workout, you can only expect 50 percent results. I cannot emphasize enough the importance of believing in yourself. Do not let anyone tell you whether or not you can accomplish something. I have fought adversity all my life, but the driving force that has kept me going is the realization that the mind is a powerful tool. Positive thinking along with the right goals in proper perspective will keep you on track. Keep trying to visualize yourself succeeding in the Master Level. Visualization will allow your body to reach levels that require much more than just sheer determination.

I am a strong believer in the family, and sometimes we must sacrifice personal desires for proper priorities. It is easy to get caught up in the trivial and vain things of life and forget what is most important. I believe we should keep ourselves physically fit so that the quality of life with our family allows us to enjoy it. Don't go so overboard in your pursuit of excellence that your family or friends forget who you are or what you look like. You may look good, but if you lose the people whom you love in the process, is it worth it?

So work hard to improve your quality of life and try sharing the Master Level with other members of your family or friends. Having a partner to be accountable to helps in motivation and support. Use every tool, asset, and support mechanism you have available to you to be successful. Adding these tools along with proper goals and motivation that comes from within, and you have the keys to succeed in the Master Level and in life.

" I believe we should keep ourselves physically fit so that the quality of life with our family allows us to enjoy it. "

Unleash Your Greatness

AT BRONZE BOW PUBLISHING WE ARE COMMITTED to helping you achieve your **ultimate potential** in functional athletic strength, fitness, natural muscular development, and all-around superb health and youthfulness.

Our books, videos, newsletters, Web sites, and training seminars will bring you the very latest in scientifically validated information that has been carefully extracted and compiled from leading scientific, medical, health, nutritional, and fitness journals worldwide.

Our goal is to empower you! To arm you with the best possible knowledge in all facets of strength and personal development so that you can make the right choices that are appropriate for *you*.

Now, as always, **the difference between greatness and mediocrity** begins with a choice. It is said that knowledge is power. But that statement is a half truth. Knowledge is power only when it has been tested, proven, and applied to your life. At that point knowledge becomes wisdom, and in wisdom there truly is *power.* The power to help you choose wisely.

So join us as we bring you the finest in health-building information and natural strength-training strategies to help you reach your ultimate potential.

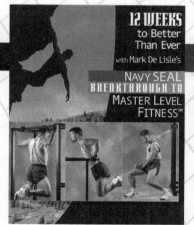

12 Weeks to Better Than Ever

MARK DE LISLE'S DAILY WORKOUT GUIDE to his *Navy SEAL Breakthrough to Master Level Fitness*™. Everything you need to know to reshape, reenergize, revitalize, and renew every muscle in your body from head to toe in 12 weeks or less.

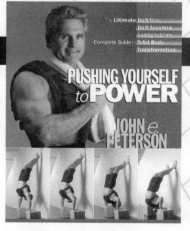

Pushing Yourself to Power

BY JOHN E. PETERSON

IF TARZAN WERE ALIVE TODAY, THIS IS THE WORKOUT HE'D FOLLOW. This is the ultimate, complete guide to total body transformation from a 50-year-old businessman/physical fitness expert who has a physique that makes eighteen-year-olds jealous. Guaranteed to turn lambs into lions! Do it now! Do it anywhere! And best of all—you'll never have to buy another gym membership or another piece of equipment unless you want to!

FOR INFORMATION ON ALL OUR EXCITING NEW SPORTS AND FITNESS PRODUCTS, CONTACT:

BRONZE BOW PUBLISHING
2600 East 26th Street
Minneapolis, MN 55406

WEB SITES
www.bronzebowpublishing.com
www.masterlevelfitness.com

612.724.8200   Toll Free **866.724.8200**   FAX **612.724.8995**